THE LUPUS SOLUTION

Your Step-By-Step Functional Medicine Guide to Understanding Lupus, Avoiding Flares, and Achieving Long-Term Remission

**Dr. Tiffany Caplan
and Dr. Brent Caplan**

This book is dedicated to you

This book is dedicated to our amazing family and friends; your support has helped us spread the message of hope to so many people. To our patients and clients, your successes are an inspiration to others and give us the power, motivation, and wisdom to continue to change lives every day. And to those battling autoimmunity and lupus, never give up hope. This book is for everyone who wants to better understand this mysterious disease and learn how remission is possible. This book is for you.

A Word from the Doctors Behind
The Lupus Solution

Many people, including doctors, see a lupus diagnosis as a life sentence, something that only gets worse with time and has to be managed for the rest of their life, however long that may be. After years of helping people with autoimmune conditions like lupus go into remission, we have witnessed healing and know this doesn't have to be the case. Thousands of people have successfully put their autoimmunity into remission and are living happy, healthy lives without fear of impending complications, and you can too.

While knowledge is powerful, it is only as powerful as the actions you take with it. Our goal is to educate people with lupus, teaching them what they need to know to put their disease into remission and sharing simple steps they can take to start healing today. We only have one body, and without our health, what do we really have? We all deserve health, and that starts with understanding what is going on in our body, so we can take control of our health.

Supporting a Loved One with Lupus

Lupus sufferers need the support of their loved ones. The diagnosis can be a lonely and terrifying one, even for those surrounded by loved ones. It is hard, even for the most supportive loved ones, to fully understand what they are facing and the day-to-day struggles and challenges they go through. Autoimmunity is invisible for the most part, making it hard to see just by looking at someone, and a lot of the pain and suffering is often hidden and difficult to cope with.

If you know or love someone with lupus, this book will give you a better understanding of not only what challenges they face, but also how you can better support them and help them on their health journey. The path to health isn't always straight or smooth sailing and requires dedication and motivation, which is why having a good support system can play a large role in overall health outcomes. Just by having a better overall understanding of what lupus is and how it impacts health, you can better support someone through it, be their cheerleader, and have a positive impact on their chance of recovery.

Additionally, you can choose to go through the healing journey with them. Even if you are not personally struggling with an autoimmune disease yourself, everyone can make positive changes in their life that can help optimize their full potential, whether that is gaining more energy, losing weight, or just preventing future health issues. This book can help you identify areas of your own health that can be improved, and you can support your loved one on their health journey by making changes with them.

Why Lupus?

After Dr. Tiffany found out a family member was diagnosed with lupus after years of struggling with mysterious symptoms and being labeled with everything from depression to fibromyalgia, she realized the need for help and hope for those suffering with this life-altering disease.

I realized that while we were successfully helping people with lupus achieve remission in our practice, the public generally believed you couldn't do anything for lupus, which couldn't be further from the truth. We were seeing people taken off drugs they were prescribed for the rest of their lives and seeing them regaining their health and getting their life back, and we realized that we needed to share that lupus remission is possible.

So she and her partner and husband, Dr. Brent Caplan, started Caplan Health Institute and The Lupus Solution to better educate those diagnosed with lupus and their loved ones about this devastating disease and to give hope for answers and safe, natural solutions.

Lupus is becoming more and more prevalent and is often misdiagnosed. Our team has helped coach people around the world through the necessary changes to regain their health and put their autoimmunity in remission.

Everyone deserves health and that begins with understanding the root cause and what your body needs to be healthy.

We have people reaching out to us daily, asking how they can regain their health. The diagnosis of lupus does not have to be a life sentence. It is the opportunity to take control of your health and learn how you too can join the thousands of people that we have helped successfully reverse their health conditions and regain their lives. You deserve to feel like yourself again and be in control of your own body.

A better future begins today!

For more information and additional resources, check out caplanhealthinstitute.com.

Nearly two-thirds of Americans between the ages of 18–34 have either not heard about lupus or know little or nothing about lupus beyond the name. This is particularly disturbing because this is the age group at greatest risk for the disease.

Table of Contents

PART ONE

The Foundation

CHAPTER ONE

The Facts/Understanding Lupus

The Lupus Story

All too often we get patients coming in with the same health story. And after suffering for years and trying just about everything out there, a lot of times we are their final hope. Out of all the different types of patients that we see, people struggling with autoimmune conditions such as lupus tend to be the most frustrated. And honestly, they have every right to be. For many dealing with an autoimmune disease, it is a very long and frustrating battle to find help and get answers. And sometimes this battle goes on for years before even getting diagnosed and having a name for what is plaguing them. This struggle is often long and mentally, emotionally, and physically draining and can lead to loss of hope and complacency. The good news is, it doesn't have to be this way, and we want to show you how.

For most people, they can remember a point in their life when things started to change, when their health made a turn for the worse. At one point they start to notice abnormal symptoms. Maybe they are tired for no reason or have joint pain for no reason, or maybe they just feel a little depressed and not like themselves. These changes are usually gradual and can be traced back to a stressful event or time in their life. For others, symptoms start more suddenly and sometimes seem to come out of nowhere. One day they're fine and the next they are waking up with pain or a rash with no apparent cause. Most symptoms start off small. Maybe you notice your knee acting up while walking upstairs, or maybe you start having a hard time getting through the day like you used to or gaining weight without changing anything you're doing. These seemingly small symptoms are the first signs your body is trying to use to tell you that something is wrong. The problem is, most people and their doctors don't take them seriously until they start to get worse.

One challenge most people with autoimmunity face is the fact that autoimmunity is essentially invisible, meaning you can't necessarily tell someone has something wrong just by looking at them. Lupus is one such disease. Besides the hallmark "butterfly rash" some people with lupus get, most signs or symptoms are internal and can't be seen by just looking at someone. This poses a challenge for not only the doctor, but also the person experiencing the symptoms as it is sometimes hard to explain what exactly they are experiencing.

Besides being invisible, lupus also affects people differently, adding another layer of challenge to proper diagnosis. We have seen firsthand the struggles they face and the frustrations they deal with. In this book we hope to shed some light for people dealing with this devastating disease and show them a better path to a brighter future where they can not only restore their health but regain their life.

The diagnosis of lupus is not to be taken lightly. Lupus is a serious disease typically involving and affecting many parts and systems of the body and leading to many serious and sometimes life-threatening complications. Like many other autoimmune conditions, symptoms tend to come on gradually, so it may take the person years to recognize their symptoms are abnormal and sometimes many more years for them to finally receive the diagnosis and have an answer for what is plaguing them.

Life-threatening conditions can develop rapidly, and patients need to be monitored closely and often for any changes. Functional laboratory testing can offer hope and a window into monitoring and catching changes before complications set in.

What Is Lupus?

In order to really answer what lupus is, we need to dive into what makes lupus unique and really come to understand the "why" of the problem so we may find a solution. A majority of people with lupus (over 63 percent) report being incorrectly diagnosed, and half report seeing four or more different healthcare providers for their symptoms before being diagnosed.

So why does this happen?
And what can we do about it?

Systemic lupus erythematosus (SLE or lupus for short) is a life-altering, multisystem autoimmune disease. In fact, lupus is not just *one disease*. Since it can affect many different body parts (skin, joints, and/or organs) and present with a wide range of symptoms and complications—many of which are potentially fatal—no two people with lupus have the same exact disease process. They can deal with a variety of different and sometimes seemingly unrelated issues, which makes lupus unique *and* hard to treat and diagnose.

Lupus is not a cancer or an infection; rather it is an underlying problem with the person's own immune system, causing it to go haywire and attack the person's own body, *which it is obviously not supposed to do.* Known as "the great imitator," the symptoms can vary and mimic many other conditions and diseases. You cannot "catch" lupus from someone who has it, but you could have a genetic predisposition to it if it runs in your family.

Lupus not only decreases quality of life by creating various symptoms, such as skin rashes, pain, and fatigue, but it can also impact overall life expectancy, leading to life-threatening complications or early death.

Unfortunately, due to the complexity of lupus, the standard of care outcomes are less than ideal. People are being told that the diagnosis in itself is almost a life sentence: an incurable and potentially life-threatening disease, riddled with life-limiting symptoms and little hope for relief. The only small relief is taking numerous medications accompanied by more and more side effects. Lupus, just like many other chronic diseases, is viewed as a chronic, progressive, degenerative disease that is expected to get worse with time. Since this is what many doctors are led to believe—and unfortunately due to standard of care treatment of lupus, tend to see—their experience with treating this disease tends to further perpetuate and confound this lack of hope.

As you will learn in this book, the standard of care treatment of lupus falls short. But there is hope for lupus! Thousands of people have successfully put their autoimmunity into remission and have regained their lives. But in order to solve a problem such as lupus, you first have to understand the problem.

Lupus is a complex disease, but sometimes the simple changes you can make on a daily basis can change your course and lead you down the path to finally managing your immune system and ridding yourself of the symptoms that stand in your way of living your best life. The standard path of lupus is one of pain and suffering, and in order to get different results, you have to do something different. Everyone deserves health and the chance to control their destiny.

Different Types of Lupus

The general term *lupus* refers to **SLE**; however, there are multiple forms of lupus under the greater umbrella of diagnosis. While a majority of cases have systemic involvement and affect multiple body parts or organ systems, some forms of lupus affect only a specific tissue, such as the skin. And while most forms of lupus tend to have lifelong implications, some forms cause only temporary or short-term effects.

Neonatal Lupus

Neonatal lupus refers to the development of lupus in a newborn who is born to a mother that has lupus. This is a rare disease when the mother's lupus antibodies affect the developing fetus, leading to rashes and/or heart damage.

Cutaneous Lupus

Cutaneous lupus refers to the involvement of the skin. This can occur with or without the systemic form of lupus (SLE). Roughly

10 percent of lupus cases solely affect the skin without other systemic involvement. The classic example of cutaneous lupus is the symbolic butterfly rash across the nose and cheeks. Around 25 percent of people with the systemic form, SLE, will also have skin involvement.

Discoid Lupus

Discoid lupus refers to a type of cutaneous lupus that causes disc-shaped rashes that most commonly affect the head, face, and ears. These round rashes can cause permanent discoloration of the skin and damage to the hair follicles. When discoid lupus affects the scalp, it can cause areas of irreversible hair loss. Fortunately, most people with chronic discoid lupus do not develop the systemic form.

Drug-Induced Lupus

Drug-induced lupus refers to a syndrome that presents as SLE, but as the name suggests, it is caused by a reaction to certain medications. Drug-induced lupus can present clinically identical to SLE, but the symptoms go away once stopping the medication that caused it.

What Is Autoimmunity?

Lupus is an autoimmune disease in the same category as conditions such as rheumatoid arthritis, multiple sclerosis, and psoriasis.

The word *autoimmune* can be broken down into two parts: auto, meaning "self," and immune, meaning the immune system. Autoimmune refers to the immune system's attack on self-tissue. Or in other words, your body's system designed to protect you and fight off infections actually starts to attack your own organs, tissues, cells, or cell components, part of your own body. Having your body attack itself is obviously not normal. So why does this happen? And more importantly, what can we do about it? Just like with any problem in life, in order to fix it, you first have to understand what it is and why is it happening, which we dive further into throughout this book.

ANA *(Antinuclear Antibody)*

One of the common lab findings for lupus is a marker called antinuclear antibody, or ANA. ANA is a marker that shows your immune system has attacked your own cell nucleus, which houses your DNA, the genetic information that makes up your body. In order for ANA to be positive, at one point your immune system had to be exposed to your cell nucleus, which lives within your cells, and in order for your immune system to be exposed to it and cause an attack, your cells had to have broken apart and "spilled out" their contents. Because the insides of your cells are never supposed to be floating around outside your cells, your immune system views them as foreign and attacks them as a safety mechanism. Once your immune system "tags" your nucleus contents as being "bad," if it ever sees that material again, it will deem it harmful and attempt to destroy it.

Cell nuclear material is, of course, in all your cells; therefore, if or when you experience tissue destruction in any part of your body, say your skin, and your immune system gets exposed to that "harmful" nuclear material again, it can attack it and anything that looks like it. This can lead to the autoimmune attack against your skin cells, such as the malar butterfly rash with lupus. Just like if the immune system encounters nuclear material in your joints, it can then cause an attack in the joints, causing pain and inflammation. This is part of the reason lupus is such a complex disease that involves multiple body tissues, parts, and systems. This is also a reason it can make diagnosis and treatment that much harder. And yet another reason why the person with lupus needs to be viewed and treated as a whole and not just lumped into a bunch of different medical specialties and viewed as having a bunch of separate problems. Autoimmunity is a puzzle, and putting all the pieces together effectively makes all the difference in recovery and makes remission possible.

Autoimmunity: The Perfect Storm

Getting diagnosed with an autoimmune disease is somewhat like being hit by the perfect storm. In general, in order for your immune system to essentially turn on you, something has to make it do so. In functional medicine, there is an equation of sorts we like to use:

---

genetic predisposition + *trigger* + *leaky gut* = *autoimmunity*

In other words, a perfect storm of things have to line up to cause your immune system to start mistaking parts of your own body as being bad.

While we know most of your immune system starts to form the day you are born, new emerging research shows that your immune system may even begin to form before you are born. This means that even things such as being born via C-section instead of vaginally or being bottle fed versus breastfed can impact your immune system. Your mother's health plays a major role as well as your inherit antibodies (your immune system's memory cells), which come from your mother's breastmilk.

It appears that children born to mothers with autoimmunity tend to have a higher risk of developing autoimmunity themselves. This is where genetics come into play. You can have a higher chance of developing an autoimmune disease just because it runs in your family. However, this book covers emerging information from the field of research called epigenetics, or the study of how we can influence our genes through diet and lifestyle. As we are learning, we have the ability to "turn off" bad genes and "turn on" good ones by things we do on a regular basis. So just because you have autoimmunity in your family doesn't mean you are destined to develop it, but if you do, it also doesn't mean you have to live with it either.

The next part to the equation is a trigger, or something that sets off the problem. We like to think that triggering disease in our body is like a gunshot. Our genes load the gun, but something in our environment or lifestyle creates a stress that pulls the trigger when it comes to chronic disease. We will be going into depth on the eight common triggers that perpetuate autoimmunity and exploring how to identify and address each one as it pertains to your body. These triggers could be things like infections, stressful events, and hormone changes or imbalances.

A common trigger for women is pregnancy, which in itself is not only stressful on the body but is also the perfect timing of a hormonal change and an immune system shift that can influence our genes. Puberty and menopause also are common times for autoimmunity to be triggered in women due to hormonal fluctuations.

Another common trigger can be food. Your immune system can start to react in a negative way to the food you are eating due to something called "leaky gut." In this sense, food can be either good and provide necessary, healing nutrients to the body, or it can be giving your body the wrong messages and therefore feed disease and cause inflammation. Understanding what you should and should not be eating is critical when it comes to autoimmunity. Unfortunately, it's not as simple as a one-size-fits-all diet, and each person's body can react differently to the same foods. We will go into more detail into how you can determine the best nutrition plan for your body in later chapters.

Leaky gut is the third piece of the puzzle when it comes to developing autoimmunity. A breakdown of the barriers that protect you from the outside world is the perfect opportunity for your immune system to be upregulated. This central area of dysfunction is at the core of most autoimmune disease. We will discuss the reasons behind this as well as how you can heal leaky gut later on.

And inflammation. We can't forget the root of all chronic disease: inflammation.

But the first thing to understand about inflammation is that not all inflammation is bad. In fact, inflammation is your body's natural response to what it perceives as a harm or stress, and at the root is actually a healing mechanism. However, when inflammation becomes chronic or doesn't go away, it becomes harmful and not only perpetuates dysfunction in the body and contributes to symptoms like pain, but it also can keep your immune system in overdrive and be a major factor in perpetuating autoimmunity.

Inflammation can show up in the body in symptoms such as pain, brain fog, and depression. It can come from things like your diet and environment, but also hidden things like blood sugar issues or hormonal imbalances that sometimes don't show up with symptoms right away or are harder to identify. We will discuss how to identify inflammation in your body later and what you can do to combat and avoid it.

Overall, inflammation is an underlying factor in most chronic conditions and can trigger and or perpetuate an autoimmune condition. Understanding inflammation, what is causing it, and how to stop it are important steps in learning how to heal and how to put autoimmune conditions like lupus in remission.

Now that you know a little more about what autoimmunity is, we will be diving into how the immune system works in future chapters so we can better understand how the system that is supposed to protect us can turn on us.

Complications

Infections are the leading cause of death in patients with SLE. People with autoimmune diseases can become severely ill from simple and common infections such as the flu. This is in part due to the involvement of the immune system in lupus but also due to the prescribed medications. Many of the drugs used to manage autoimmune conditions are immunosuppressants, which suppress the immune system.

In lupus, like many other autoimmune conditions, the immune system is actually overactive; therefore, the treatment in the standard drug model is to simply suppress it. But as you can guess, when you suppress the immune system, other issues can arise. Your immune system is meant to protect you, and by essentially shutting it down, you create the perfect opportunity for a whole host of other infectious agents, which we normally get exposed to and fight off daily, to infect you and make you sick. And without a healthy immune system to fight those off, people with lupus are more susceptible to poor health outcomes and complications due to infection.

Even people who are not on immunosuppressants face challenges with infections and their body's ability to fight them off. Even though the immune system is *overactive* in autoimmunity, it doesn't mean it is good at fighting off infections. Our immune system is like a balancing scale that works when each side is able to stay balanced with the other, and in autoimmunity, this balance shifts, causing problems with your immune system's ability to successfully maintain its normal functions. We will talk more about immune balance later.

Other serious complications of lupus involve renal failure and central nervous system (CNS) involvement. Many people with lupus are diagnosed and suffer the consequences of poor kidney function. Our kidneys are important organs that not only help eliminate waste from our body through urine production, but also help us absorb nutrients, help control our blood pressure, and make sure our cells are getting oxygen and nutrients to function. As previously mentioned, a majority of the time, kidney dysfunction goes on for years without being diagnosed or caught early enough when it can still be prevented. This can lead to other complications and symptoms in the body that can appear as if they are coming from somewhere else. Something like high blood pressure can be thought of as just a cardiovascular marker when in fact it could be stemming from an underlying kidney dysfunction. If we monitor and catch things early, not only can we minimize symptoms, but we can also help prevent life-threatening complications such as renal failure.

Heart disease is another leading cause of death in people with lupus. In fact, according to Johns Hopkins, "the risk of heart attack in women with lupus aged 35–44 is 50-times greater than that of women without lupus, and for everyone with lupus the risk is increased 7- to 9-fold."

Stroke and heart attacks are common and serious complications of the vascular effects from SLE as well as septic arthritis. Autoimmune destruction and inflammation caused by lupus are known to affect the heart and cardiovascular system. People on immunosuppressants have an even higher risk of inflammation of the heart, or myocarditis, due to a decreased ability to fight off infections that commonly cause myocarditis. When lupus affects the cardiovascular system, it can lead to symptoms such as:

- Shortness of breath

- Chest pain

- Unexplained rapid or irregular heartbeats

- High blood pressure

People with lupus often have symptoms that are not specific to lupus. These include fever, fatigue, weight loss, blood clots, and hair loss in spots or around the hairline. They may also have heartburn, stomach pain, and poor circulation to the fingers and toes. Pregnant women can have miscarriages.

Don't ignore symptoms! As we will discuss later, symptoms, as benign as they may sometimes seem, are your early warning signals. Symptoms are how your body tries to communicate with you that something is wrong. Never dismiss what your body is trying to say as unimportant. Listening to your symptoms might just save your life.

When we look for the root cause of the problem and ask, *Why did this happen in the first place?* and *What is causing it to continue?*, then, and only then, can we resolve the true problem at the core instead of merely managing it. This is the beauty of functional medicine and our personalized approach to addressing lupus.

Epidemiology of Lupus

According to the National Resource Center on Lupus, more than 16,000 new cases of lupus are reported every year in the United States alone. It is estimated that at least 1.5 million Americans suffer from it, and the rates may be higher due to many people who remain undiagnosed. Worldwide, lupus affects approximately over 5 million people, and diagnosis rates continue to rise.

Lupus is two to three times more prevalent among women of color—African Americans, Hispanics/Latinos, Asians, Native Americans, and Pacific Islanders—than among Caucasian women. Recent research indicates that lupus affects about 1 in 537 young African American women. And African American lupus patients are more likely to have organ system involvement, more serious complications, and higher rates of mortality.

People age eighteen to thirty-four are the highest risk demographic for developing SLE. And yet over 72 percent of eighteen-to-thirty-four-year-olds have never heard of or know little of lupus beyond the name. The lack of public information and awareness on lupus may be a factor in the struggle to get accurately diagnosed.

With lupus, many times, multiple tissues, organs, or systems are affected, and the symptoms aren't always easy to connect the dots or pinpoint the problem. Because patients can present with a wide array of symptoms that don't seem to be connected, healthcare providers may think multiple different diseases or conditions are present simultaneously when in fact, the symptoms may be able to all be traced back to "the great imitator": lupus. This may contribute to the reason it takes on average over seven years and four different healthcare providers to come to the diagnosis of lupus.

One in three people diagnosed with lupus also suffer from multiple other autoimmune diseases. Other common autoimmune diseases include Sjogren's and Hashimoto's. Sjogren's affects the mucus membranes of places such as the eyes, mouth, and nose. People with Sjogren's experience extreme dryness in those areas, which can lead to other issues. Hashimoto's is an autoimmune disease that causes an attack and destruction of the thyroid gland leading to symptoms of hypothyroid or low thyroid. Symptoms of low thyroid include things like fatigue, insomnia, hair loss, constipation, and depression. Many symptoms associated with autoimmune diagnosis can overlap, thus making it that much harder to pinpoint the cause of the symptoms and causing doctors to just chase the symptoms with medications.

Cost of Lupus

Managing autoimmune diagnoses costs the United States over $100 billion annually. A 2008 study published in *Arthritis & Rheumatology* found that a lupus patient's healthcare costs average $12,000 annually. The study also found that the mean annual productivity costs (lost hours of productive work) for employed lupus patients is $8,000. Thus, the mean annual total costs to a lupus patient is $20,000. And this doesn't just go away since it is a chronic disease. Unfortunately, these costs leave the person in the same place year after year as the mainstream treatment approach is limited and aimed at simply minimizing symptoms, many times by suppressing the immune system, instead of actually treating or fixing the disease.

Two of three lupus patients report a complete or partial loss of income due to inability to work full time because of disease complications. The chronic fatigue alone accounts for loss in daily function and productivity. Not to mention the other symptoms, such as pain and depression, that wreak havoc on the ability to get through the day let alone keep up with the hectic demands of work and everyday life. Many of our patients have suffered financial hardship due to the effects of lupus, not only in the costs of disease management and expensive and ineffective drugs but also lost wages and even having to go on disability due to inability to hold a stable job.

The cost not only comes with financial burden but also the physical and mental emotional cost of living with a disease you are led to believe will take your life. The loss of hope is possibly the most devastating part. Feeling helpless leads people to give up, and giving up makes it impossible to move forward and change. If all you get from this book is this, please don't give up. There is hope for recovery and remission and potential to regain your life no matter your age or stage of life. Thousands have successfully followed this path and are living happy, healthy, fulfilling lives, and you can too. Don't let lupus win.

Healing Is a Journey

Many suffering from lupus would agree that while symptoms such as pain and fatigue have a negative impact on their daily lives, the frustration that comes with this disease may far outweigh the physical symptoms. A lot of the frustration stems from misunderstanding the disease as a whole. Most people are diagnosed after years of suffering from a wide array of different seemingly unrelated symptoms. Many times, these people have been repeatedly told their labs are normal and there is nothing wrong, leading them to believe that their symptoms are "normal"—simply a result of age or stress.

But they are not normal. Once you receive your diagnosis, you can heal by committing to the lifestyle changes outlined in this book. Healing is a journey and will take some changes on your part. Don't give up. The long-term benefits of making necessary changes far outweigh the short-term hardship of making those changes. And the more you practice better habits, the better you feel and the easier it becomes.

It's important to understand that there is no quick fix or fad diet that can lead to long-term results. It is a lifestyle change that needs to be followed lifelong and requires learning what that means for your body.

Yet sometimes creating new habits can be hard. Changing things takes time and patience. Even though it seems like the diagnosis happens overnight, many health conditions take years if not decades in the making to get to the point they can be diagnosed.

This means your body was experiencing these symptoms for a while, and so it will take time to fix it. The body can only compensate for dysfunction so long before things aren't working like they should, and symptoms start to show up.

While receiving your diagnosis is frustrating, the even more frustrating part is a lack of understanding from loved ones, friends, and even doctors. When you have a systemic autoimmune disease that can attack random tissues in your body and your symptoms show up as a whole range of seemingly unrelated issues, not only is it hard to explain what you are dealing with, but it is also hard for others to relate and even harder to get the correct diagnosis in a timely manner. How do you explain to someone how it feels to feel your body falling apart when they have never experienced anything similar before? That lack of understanding can seem isolating and one of the hardest parts of being diagnosed.

For the Loved Ones of Those with Lupus

How to help support someone you love who has lupus:

- Try to understand what they are going through on a regular basis and how it impacts their daily life.

- Offer to help with tasks that may be difficult when they aren't feeling well, such as helping out around the house or in the workplace.

- Encourage healthy eating habits and follow them yourself.

- Encourage healthy lifestyle habits such as going for a walk or going to bed at a good time.

- Listen—be an ear for when they need to talk and a hug when they need it.

- And just be there for them. We all need some help sometimes, and creating a support team can make their health journey that much easier and successful.

Imagine stepping into their shoes for a day and feeling the pain, fatigue, or other symptoms they are dealing with. If you've never experienced anything like that, remember a time you had the flu or something similar and the exhaustion, aches, and foggy mind that came with being sick. People with lupus live with this on a daily basis. It can feel like their body is falling apart and can be mentally, emotionally, and physically draining. Having someone understand how much this impacts their daily life can help them not feel so alone, which by itself takes a toll on someone's ability to heal.

Along with feeling empathy, you can make changes alongside them during their healing journey. Even if you yourself are not suffering from any ailments or chronic health issues, it can be beneficial for you too to learn about yourself, your body, and how to live a healthier life. It's never too early or too late to create healthier habits and help promote health and prevention.

So many times our patients' spouses or significant others participated in making changes in their life as well, and more often than not, the spouse experienced positive health outcomes they didn't even know they needed or could have! Many times, we get so used to how we feel on a regular basis that it seems "normal" when in fact we are experiencing symptoms and problems that we just don't notice, but they are our body's way of telling us something is wrong and needs to change. A lot of times we also accept what is common as being normal and make excuses like "It's just age," "I'm just getting older," or "Everyone feels tired sometimes," and we write off symptoms as something we just deal with or get used to them. So just because you feel "fine" doesn't mean you can't feel better or perhaps even prevent future problems from coming on and causing problems later on.

Those of you who are suffering with lupus need to let your loved ones in. Let's face it, sometimes change is hard! But so is being sick. Living day to day in fear and frustration and being weighed down by pain or fatigue can make even simple daily tasks near impossible, and doing them on your own only makes it that much harder.

Having people in your life to help guide and encourage you along the way can have a huge impact on your success and overall health outcomes.

Ignorance may be bliss, but what you don't know may kill you. Knowledge can be a powerful tool—if you know how to use it. In the following chapters, we will be explaining what lupus is at the core to better help you and your loved ones understand this mysterious disease and then will teach you how to implement necessary changes to work toward the goal of remission and optimal health.

Tip: Note down anything that resonates with you as you go through this book to help guide you through personalizing this approach for your health goals and what you would like to achieve. One of the simplest and most powerful tools you have available to you is a pen. Writing things down helps you better learn and understand and helps you remember and organize this new information.

Side Story from Dr. Tiffany:
My Journey to Health and Happiness

Looking back, one of the best experiences in my life was having survived my low. My own personal health journey got me to where I am today and drives my passion for helping others as I was helped. I thank functional medicine for saving my life and helping me find my purpose. Having been diagnosed with severe depression and anxiety in grad school completely changed me. My mood, brain fog, fatigue, and lack of motivation was not only affecting my life and causing me to struggle in school for the first time but was also affecting the people around me. My then boyfriend, now husband, Brent, was constantly afraid I would hurt myself as I had opened up to him about wanting to, and I realized the emotional toll it was taking on him and our relationship. Getting to a place where I finally recognized that this feeling was not normal and something needed to change, I started on the path to finding health and happiness.

Looking back, that time in my life was one of the hardest things I've been through but also one of the biggest blessings as I am now able to help so many more people because of what I experienced. It helped me realize how isolating yourself while dealing with health issues can be damaging. I didn't let anyone in for a long time because I didn't want to put that burden on them, but I also didn't know how to really explain or help them understand what I was going through either. The more I tried to push others away, the worse I felt. If it weren't for the love and support of Brent and my family, I wouldn't be here today. My health journey not only taught me a lot about myself and healthy living but also about the healing process itself and how important it is to have that support along the way. The road to health isn't always easy or straightforward, and life is always going to interfere, but with a little help and guidance, anything is possible!

Nicole's Story

Lupus was affecting every aspect of Nicole's life when she came to see us. She was diagnosed with SLE and Sjogren's a few years before coming in but had been struggling with various health ailments on and off since she was thirty. And now at forty-eight years old, she was living with the devastating diagnosis of autoimmunity.

She came in complaining of extreme fatigue; dry eyes and mouth; frequent, severe headaches; joint pain; brain fog; insomnia; and hair loss. She had been experiencing weird symptoms on and off for over a decade but until a few years ago didn't have a name for what was plaguing her. Concerned with how her symptoms were getting worse despite medical treatment, she worried she would be hospitalized again. She was also concerned since her mother had also been diagnosed with lupus and developed and passed away from complications of multiple sclerosis, another autoimmune condition. She wanted to prevent developing further complications or autoimmunity herself.

She was seeing a rheumatologist for her lupus and joint pains, a neurologist for her headaches, a cardiologist for her past history of chest pains in her thirties, and her primary care physician. She was taking Prednisone and Plaquenil, both immunosuppressants, for her lupus; alprazolam for sleep and anxiety; fluoxetine for depression; Benadryl for allergies and to help her fall asleep; and ibuprofen for pain. Despite taking her meds, she was still constantly fatigued, in pain, and missing work due to debilitating days-long headaches. She only could go to work a couple of days a week and then was wiped out for days after.

No longer able to even enjoy her hobbies or social activities outside of work, because she never knew when symptoms would get in the way, she was sad and frustrated that her life was being run by her condition and didn't know if she could be helped but was tired of feeling sick and tired and was ready for change. Her story will be continued throughout the book.

CHAPTER TWO

Gathering Information

Lupus Diagnosis

Most autoimmune diseases typically need to cause enough damage before the symptoms even start, and a certain amount of destruction and symptomatology needs to occur before diagnosis.

This is a problem since it can sometimes take months for the symptoms to even be noticed as a sign that something is wrong. Unless there is a very sudden triggering event or onset of a severe symptom, this disease tends to remain nearly invisible for months or years before the person feels concerned enough to seek medical help. One of the first signs may be symptoms of Raynaud's, which causes the tips of the fingers or toes to turn white when cold, or perhaps some mild achiness in the joints. These seemingly small, nonimportant symptoms tend to be ignored or thought of as "normal" until they continue to persist or worsen as the underlying disease worsens. At this point, with minimal symptoms, it will not be obviously lupus so typically it will be misdiagnosed. Often lupus is identified as "undifferentiated connective tissue disease."

Knowing this, you need to be proactive. Many complications don't happen overnight, and in fact, sometimes they can take years to manifest. The first sign of a heart attack is often sudden death. Why wait for the complication to come on when you can identify you are heading there before the damage sets in and can't be reversed?

Monitoring signs of inflammation and underlying dysfunction in the body before the problems set in offers better hope for fixing and preventing debilitating or life-threatening problems.

Even if you monitor your systems and recognize that something is wrong earlier on, many doctors check only a limited number of lab markers associated with the particular symptoms or systems that the person is experiencing issues in. This creates an issue with catching things early and before the complications worsen. Appropriate and thorough testing is essential in treating and managing lupus and needs to cover a wide look at the body as a whole instead of different pieces or parts. To get full testing, you can turn to functional medicine. Functional lab testing and evaluation go above and beyond the standard markers and allow a deeper look at what is going on in all systems of the body to view the interconnected web that makes up the whole person. We know the body does not operate as a bunch of separate and individual body parts or systems, so why are we being tested and treated as if we are?

Lupus diagnosis is based on multiple criteria, and standard guidelines have been set for requirements for diagnosis. Diagnosis is based on two main components: symptoms or clinical presentation and laboratory findings. In order for lupus to be diagnosed, a minimum of four out of eleven criteria must be present. The more positive criteria, the more confident the diagnosis. There are "clinical criteria" and "immunologic criteria," and in order to diagnose lupus, a person must meet at least one criterion in each of those two classifications as part of the minimum. It is possible to have lupus and not have four or more of the diagnosis criteria. Then again, someone with another condition such as rheumatoid arthritis can meet the criteria and not have lupus. The criteria are good guidelines but are not always 100 percent of the picture.

The 11 Diagnosis Criteria	
Clinical Criteria	1. Malar/cheek rash
	2. Discoid rash
	3. Photosensitivity
	4. Ulcerations of oral mucosa
	5. Joint pain and inflammation not attributed to other disease or trauma
	6. Serositis: Inflammation of the serous tissues, which line the lungs, heart, inner lining of the abdomen, and associated organs (can cause chest pain when breathing deeply)
	7. Renal disease (any of the following): >3+ proteinuria, cellular casts, proteinuria >.5 grams per day
	8. CNS involvement: seizures or psychosis without other cause
	9. Hematologic abnormalities (any of the following): hemolytic anemia, leucopenia (45%), lymphopenia, thrombocytopenia (30%), anemia of chronic disease
Immunologic Criteria	10. Positive ANA
	11. Additional serologic tests (any of the following): -Positive LE cell prep -Anti-native DNA antibody (50%) -Anti-Sm antibody (20%) -False-positive test for syphilis (25%)

Definitions of Above Criteria

Malar Rash

- The classic "butterfly rash," which typically covers the cheeks and bridge of the nose; is seen in only less than half of all lupus patients

Discoid Rash

- A red rash with raised coin-shaped patches that tend to get worse when exposed to sunlight

Photosensitivity

- Increased sensitivity to the sun and formation of rashes on sun-exposed areas

Ulcerations of Oral Mucosa

- Sores in the mouth or nose that last from a few days to more than a month

Joint Pain and Inflammation

- 90 percent of lupus patients have joint pain
- Most common joints/areas affected include, but are not limited to, the hands, wrists, feet, and knees
- Tenderness and swelling

Serositis

- Inflammation of the tissues that line our organs and can cause pain with non-painful activities such as taking a deep breath

Renal Disease

- 50 percent of patients have kidney complications related to their lupus. Kidney function tends to get worse with disease flares and progression but can improve with remission.

- Kidney failure is a leading cause of death in patients with lupus

CNS Involvement

- 70 percent of lupus patients have EEG (electro-encephalogram) abnormalities

- Headaches and migraines are common symptoms

- Seizures, stroke, or psychosis (medical emergencies)

Hematologic Abnormalities

- Low blood cell counts (red, white, and/or platelets)

Positive ANA

- A blood test marker that shows antibodies to self-tissue

Positive ANA

ANA is an immune attack against your cell's nucleus-home to your genetic data, or DNA. This is particularly relevant and problematic in SLE, and it is the reason it affects so many organ systems and has the potential to cause multisystem, multiorgan problems. It can attack all cells and, depending on which tissues are involved, determine the symptoms and complications that may present. This also makes diagnosis tricky as symptoms can present as other conditions or the person may appear to have multiple autoimmune conditions concurrently.

Positive ANA alone does not mean lupus. A number of other conditions can have a positive ANA, including arthritis, scleroderma, Sjogren's syndrome, polymyositis/dermatomyositis, mixed connective tissue disease, drug-induced lupus, and autoimmune hepatitis. Certain medications can also cause a positive ANA.

Let's say you sprain your ankle, that tissue injury causes an inflammatory response, and your immune cells are brought in to "clean up the mess." Now if you have damaged cells and your immune system recognizes the "guts" of the cell, cell contents like the cell nucleus, floating around where they are not supposed to be, it assumes it is something foreign that isn't supposed to be there, so it will form an antibody (your immune system's "memory" cells) to that cell nucleus. Now your immune system is producing an ANA as a result of tissue damage and not due to an autoimmune process, such as lupus. But now let's say you have lupus or a genetic predisposition to it (like a family member with it) and you sprained your ankle. Now that tissue damage from spraining your ankle can contribute to or even set off the autoimmune disease process, and your joints are now most likely the "weak spot" in your body, and your main symptoms may likely be joint pain and inflammation. This is why it is important to get a complete look at everything going on and not just one lab test.

ANA alone is a screening test for lupus since almost all patients with lupus have a positive ANA test.

Diagnostic Tests

Anti-double-stranded DNA (anti-dsDNA) is nearly specific to lupus. About 80 percent of all lupus patients with active disease have a positive anti-dsDNA result. This marker can be useful in monitoring disease progress.

Anti-Smith (anti-Sm) is usually seen in patients who do not have positive anti-dsDNA. However, this marker is not a great indicator of monitoring disease activity like anti-dsDNA is.

Anti-U1 ribonucleoprotein (anti-RNP) can be positive in SLE but also suggests, if other autoantibodies are negative, a disease called mixed connective tissue disease (MCTD), which is characterized by lupus-, scleroderma-, and dermatomyositis-like symptoms.

Anti-Ro/SSA and anti-La/SSB antibodies suggest possible development of Sjogren's syndrome and more sun-sensitive rashes. Pregnant women with these antibodies are monitored closely as the baby is at a higher risk for developing heart issues.

Antiphospholipid antibodies (aPL) are positive in about a third of lupus patients, and about 10 percent of lupus patients may have antiphospholipid syndrome. Antiphospholipid syndrome is characterized by recurring blood clots and pregnancy complications. Several tests are used to diagnose and monitor antiphospholipid antibodies: lupus anticoagulant test, anticardiolipin, and anti-beta2glycoprotein1.

Complements C3 & C4

There's no arguing that our bodies are intelligent and self-healing. Think about the last time you got a paper cut. Did it just stay an open wound forever or did it heal on its own? One of our innate healing processes is to "clean house" or get rid of the old and/or damaged cells to repair and heal. With lupus, this self-healing and ability to "clean house" can be damaged, which is the perfect stimuli to keep the immune system overactive and can be a factor in the abnormal immune response fueling lupus. In turn, the lupus antibodies also activate this complement system; therefore, measuring these complement markers, namely C3 and C4, can help indicate the activity level of the disease and can show when someone is close to or in a flare. Decreased levels of these complement proteins are associated with increased risk of autoimmune disease as well as recurrent microbial infections and can be used to monitor disease activity.

Other Important Tests

Aside from the standard criteria for diagnosis, many other important tests can be run and monitored. These include tests for inflammation, as well as other markers of general health, to rule out or identify triggers or other issues that need to be addressed. Remember, we don't want to simply "suppress inflammation" or "suppress the immune system" or throw a Band-Aid on the symptoms. We need to find and address all dysfunctions in the body that are contributing to the problem and overall loss of immune regulation. Patients with underlying issues, such as metabolic syndrome, thyroid disease, hormonal imbalance, and anemia, need to find and address these first in order to be able to address the big picture. The body works as one integrative system, and all parts and pieces play a role in overall function or dysfunction in the body. Problems like blood sugar regulation issues contribute to overall dysfunction in the body and until addressed can make it difficult or impossible to control lupus. Below is a list of other important blood markers that should be checked and monitored accordingly.

Other Important Lab Panels
Metabolic Chemistry Panel
Urinalysis
CBC with Differentials and Platelets
Iron and Anemia Markers
Hypothyroidism and Hashimoto's
Fasting Insulin and Hemoglobin A1c
Homocysteine and MTHFR status
Hs-CRP (High Sensitivity C-Reactive Protein)
ESR (Erythrocyte Sedimentation Rate)
Fibrinogen
Complement Levels (C3 and C4)
HLA-DR2 and HLA-DR3
Celiac Testing
Syphilis VDRL
Antiphospholipid and Anticardiolipin Antibodies

Doctors may also want to perform an X-ray to check for fluid around the lungs or inflammation and/or scarring of the lung tissue. An ECG, or electrocardiogram, can check for inflammation and/or fluid around the heart. Kidney biopsies may be performed if kidney disease due to SLE is suspected. Skin biopsies of rashes are used to diagnose if a rash is from SLE.

The presence of antiphospholipid antibodies signals a raised risk for certain complications such as miscarriage or blood clots. Doctors also may measure levels of certain complement proteins (a part of the immune system) in the blood to help detect the disease and follow its progress.

It is important to note that approximately 30 percent of people with lupus test positive for syphilis without having this STI (sexually transmitted infection). The VDRL (venereal disease research laboratory) and RPR (rapid plasma reagin) tests can test false-positive in these people.

Why "Normal" Labs Don't Always Mean Normal

Many times with these routine standard of care tests, doctors are routinely and unknowingly doing a disservice by running the minimal standard blood panels. The standard routine blood panel used to include an average of twenty-seven different markers or panels to get a comprehensive look at what is going on. As the years have gone on and insurance has become stricter in what tests are considered "necessary" and standard, the average panel has now been whittled down to about five markers. An average of just five markers or panels is now considered the only necessary panel for routine follow-up, and doctors are using it as the primary checkup for your yearly physical. The problem is that the common markers being tested are simply not enough to show the full picture of what is going on. This has led to an epidemic of people going to their doctor with symptoms and leaving being told they are "normal" and their labs are fine.

The other aspect that can present problems is that the lab ranges for those markers not only vary depending on what lab you go to, but they also are usually not specific enough to see less than optimal function. Another problem with lab testing is that the lab ranges are typically very broad and don't allow for sensitivity. This all means it's just as important, if not more, that the lab results are evaluated from a functional perspective as well. Just because your lab value falls somewhere within the "normal" lab range does not necessarily mean it is normal or optimal. For example, most lab ranges do not flag your kidney function marker or GFR (glomerular filtration rate) as abnormal until it is less than sixty. In fact, a lot of labs don't even give you a number for the GFR if it is at least above sixty. However, we know that a GFR less than sixty is considered stage 3 chronic kidney disease! Why do we wait to lose half our kidney function before we start to pay attention! If we monitor the lab ranges for kidney function on a regular basis and monitor for changes, we can catch a decrease in kidney function before it gets to stage 3, and the earlier it is caught, the easier it is to reverse and prevent future complications.

Stages of chronic kidney disease:

Stage 1: GFR is 90 or above (normal) but abnormal levels of protein found in urine

Stage 2: GFR is 60–89

Stage 3: GFR is 30–59

Stage 4: GFR is 15–29

Stage 5: End stage renal disease GFR under 15

As you can see, healthy functioning kidneys should have a filtration rate (GFR) of over 90. Once you get down to < 60, you are already in stage 3 of kidney dysfunction. Stage 5 is dialysis. But most labs don't flag the GFR as abnormal until you get to under 60, which at that point you are now already in stage 3 and your kidneys need help.

Optimal functional lab ranges show where our physiology works *best*. So rather than just being "in the normal lab range," functional medicine looks for numbers indicating your body is working best in that area. For example, A1c, a marker for blood sugar regulation in the body, is a ninety-day average to see how much the blood sugar fluctuates. To be told you have diabetes, your A1c must be > 6.5 by most lab ranges. However, we know that an A1c of just over 5.6 increases your risk of complications and decreases your life span. Unfortunately, the standard of care for diabetes, which healthcare providers follow to diagnose and manage diabetes, doesn't offer any help until you are in the diabetic range, meaning you can be prediabetic (5.7–6.4) for years if not decades and be told your labs are fine until one day your A1c jumps over 6.5, and now you are told you are diabetic. The guidelines followed see diabetes, as well as the other 90 percent of diseases people are dealing with nowadays, as a chronic progressive, degenerative course that only gets worse with time, not better, and the main goal in treating chronic diseases such as diabetes and autoimmunity lies in managing symptoms versus treating disease.

Most doctors base their diagnosis on the standard lab ranges, and it is standard practice for them to wait for them to be "out of range" to even mention a problem let alone diagnose it. The point is, you can test for these things early on and monitor them over time to catch these problems and start to prevent them from progressing and causing other complications down the road.

Just like your body communicates to you that something is wrong through physical symptoms, labs, when used correctly, can signal when things aren't working optimally and can help to prevent and reverse dysfunction, thus leading to optimal health outcomes.

Using Symptoms as a Tool

Avoid making this one big mistake: *Never mistake symptoms for being "normal."*

Too many times we hear, "I'm just getting old," "It's just 'normal' aging," or "I'm just tired." But just because something is common or doesn't seem "that bad" doesn't mean it is normal. Don't forget that symptoms are your body's way of communicating that *something is wrong*. Doesn't matter how benign the symptoms may be. Many times, seemingly benign problems, like fatigue or constipation, can be just the tip of the iceberg for the real problems under the surface. High blood sugar and prediabetes are great examples of this. When the body loses its ability to regulate blood sugar, one of the most foundational functions in the human body, it impacts more than just blood sugar. The symptom may be elevated blood glucose, but that is just the tip of the iceberg as to what is really under the surface actually driving that problem. So, no matter how "simple" or "common" or "normal" a symptom might be, remember this: *symptoms are never normal.*

What Is Your Body Telling You?

While symptoms can be the worst part of dealing with a chronic disease and annoying at best, symptoms aren't "bad." Symptoms are simply the way you know something isn't right and your body is telling you how and what you need to change to get better. By learning to listen to your body and what it is trying to tell you, you can take control of your health by making choices that will positively impact your health and help you put your disease in remission.

So, let's talk about how to listen to your body. Let's start with fatigue. If you are dealing with fatigue, lack of energy, or poor sleep, or if you feel like you need to rely on stimulants like caffeine or sugar to get through your day, your body is saying it is struggling to work efficiently—whether or not it is a sign that your cells are not getting enough glucose for energy production, ATP (adenosine triphosphate, or cellular energy), oxygen, or thyroid hormone or your adrenal glands are having problems regulating cortisol, the stress hormone that plays a role in your sleep/wake cycle. Overall, a vast majority of underlying problems can contribute to loss of energy or fatigue but recognizing this lack of energy as an important symptom or sign that something is wrong or not working correctly under the surface is critical to identifying the cause and, therefore, fixing the problem.

What about pain? Joint pain is a symptom of inflammation in the joints. We know that inflammation is an underlying root cause of all chronic disease, and joint pain can be a way your body tries to alert you to the underlying inflammation. Once you identify signs of inflammation being present, you can look for possible causes of inflammation: a food you are eating, a toxin in your environment, or another stressor from your diet or lifestyle.

GATHERING INFORMATION

Once you can identify the underlying cause, you can make the appropriate changes in diet and lifestyle to address it and fix the real problem instead of just masking the symptom.

Symptom Questionnaire

Because the effects of lupus are not confined to one body part or organ and can indeed affect multiple systems and organs, symptoms of lupus tend to vary widely and differ from person to person.

While symptoms alone may not always help with diagnosis, symptoms are a very important part of the clinical picture and can help as indicators of progression and/or remission.

The following symptom chart is a good reference point for those not yet diagnosed as well as those on their journey to remission. Tracking symptoms over time can help you watch for improvements that may be gradual to track progress. As you progress on your health journey, you may find that your daily quality of life improves in increments, and you start to "redefine normal" as symptoms that were consistently frequent and/or severe begin to diminish and lessen over time until you are no longer having them. For instance, people dealing with frequent headaches start to have less severe and less frequent headaches over time, so initially maybe they were having headaches four times per week, but after a while maybe they are getting them less frequently, say once every other week, and less severe to the point of not needing to take pain medication. So, if questioned if they are still having headaches, they might say yes, but by tracking frequency and severity, they can see that they are indeed less frequent and/or less severe, both signs of improvement.

Symptoms to Look For:

- Rash on arms or face after sun exposure (not sunburn)

- Sores on roof of mouth or in nose

- Fingers or toes turn white or blue with cold exposure (cold weather or water, etc.)

- The classic malar "butterfly rash," which typically covers the cheeks and bridge of the nose

- A red rash with raised coin-shaped patches that tend to get worse when exposed to sunlight

- Increased sensitivity to the sun and formation of rashes on sun-exposed areas

- Most common joints/areas affected include, but are not limited to, the hands, wrists, feet, and knees

- Joint tenderness and swelling

- Kidney failure diagnosis—a leading cause of death in patients with lupus

- Headaches and migraines, both common symptoms

- Seizures, stroke, or psychosis (medical emergencies)

- Low blood cell counts (red, white, and/or platelets)

Signs of kidney problems:

- High blood pressure

- Swollen feet and hands

- Puffiness around your eyes

- Changes in urination (blood or foam in the urine, going to the bathroom more often at night, or pain or trouble urinating)

Clinical Symptom Checklist Tracker

0 *never have this*

1 *sometimes experience this, not severe*

2 *regularly experience this or sometimes experience this but severe*

3 *regularly experience this, severe*

4 *diagnosed with this*

_____ **Fatigue**

_____ **Trouble sleeping/insomnia**

_____ **Fever**

_____ **Joint pain**

_____ **Muscle aches**

_____ **Muscle weakness**

_____ **Tenderness or swelling**

_____ **Weight loss**

_____ **Sores in mouth or nose**

_____ **Coin-shaped or butterfly-shaped rash**

_____ **Rash after sun exposure**

_____ **Dry eyes or Sjogren's**

_____ **Chest pain when taking deep breath**

_____ **Enlarged lymph nodes**

_____ **Poor circulation in fingers and/or toes**

_____	Raynaud's syndrome
_____	Sensitive to chemicals or smells
_____	Hair loss and/or bald patches
_____	Brain fog/poor concentration
_____	Depression
_____	Anxiety
_____	Dizziness or confusion
_____	Headaches
_____	Migraines
_____	Seizures
_____	Chronic infections/get sick easily
_____	Anemia
_____	Kidney failure
Total:	

Scoring: *< 5 points = mild/remission*

5-20 point = active disease

> 20 points = current flare/severe

The Functional Medicine Approach

Most people recognize that a fever is a symptom that the body is trying to fight off an infection. But symptoms could also be things like insomnia signaling adrenal fatigue or weight gain due to hormonal imbalance. When we learn to listen to our bodies and know what they are trying to tell us, we can better make the changes in our everyday lives to help support the body with what it needs to not only treat the symptoms but also address the root cause of the problem. Just like if you want to remove a weed from your garden, you can't just cut off the top of the weed. To permanently remove the weed, you must pull it out from the root.

Functional medicine addresses the symptoms at the root. As Dr. Mark Hyman, the director of the Cleveland Clinic Center for Functional Medicine, says, "Functional Medicine is the future of medicine, available now... [It] is medicine by cause, not by symptom. Functional Medicine practitioners don't, in fact, treat disease, we treat your body's ecosystem. We get rid of the bad stuff, put in the good stuff, and because your body is an intelligent system—it does the rest."

By looking at the individual as a whole, instead of just focusing on the symptoms they are having as related to different and separate body parts, we can get a deeper look at the interconnectedness of the human body and better appreciate how seemingly unrelated issues can all come from a similar cause, or what we like to call the "root cause."

Many times, we discover that the most common underlying causes driving autoimmunity in patients have simply been overlooked in the standard medical approach due to the nature of Western medicine and the systemization of how patients with chronic diseases are looked at and managed in the standard of care. It's easy for a rheumatologist to miss an underlying hormone imbalance when all their training and expertise leads them to be more concerned with the patient's joint pain. The endocrinologist's job to be more concerned with hormones and the cardiologist's job to look at the heart. But are these things really separate?

When was the last time someone asked about your stress level or your diet or if you are noticing reactions to foods or things in your environment? All these seemingly unrelated pieces are part of a much larger puzzle, the patient as a whole. All our systems and organs and cells have to play a part in keeping us alive, and they do that by communicating with one another and relying on all the other parts (cells, tissues, organs, etc.) to do their jobs. It's like a symphony, and one squeaky horn can throw off the balance and disrupt the concert.

Redefining the Standard of Care

If modern medicine has taught us anything, it's this: *there is no one-size-fits-all approach that works for everyone.* This is extremely true for people suffering from lupus. Lupus is different for everyone because everyone has a different genetic makeup, environment, and physiology. Therefore, the treatment must be different. This presents a challenge because in order to find what works for the individual, it must be tailored to the individual.

This is the opposite of how the medical model is designed to work. Instead of tailoring the treatment for the person, it is tailored to the disease label. *A pill for an ill.* However, this causes many patients in the standard of care medical model to suffer despite doing everything their doctors tell them to, and it's not their fault and a lot of times not their doctor's fault either. It is a broken model. One that has been outdated and behind research for quite some time.

In fact, it has been shown that it takes on average seventeen years for the latest research to be used in the standard medical setting. Seventeen years! Up to twenty-five years in some cases. That's simply too long. That means that most doctors are still using the knowledge they learned in school X amount of years ago without changing with the ever-evolving research that comes out on a daily basis. Even the information taught in schools is outdated or behind the times. One of the reasons for this is how the Western medical system was designed.

One hundred years ago, the things that were killing us were infections. Things like TB and the flu were claiming lives, and ideas such as the germ theory came to be popular. The fix for most illness was a drug. Take an antibiotic for an infection. A vaccine to prevent disease. The idea was simple: x pathogen = x drug. And this worked! However, those illnesses that were the leading causes of death a hundred years ago are no longer the leading causes.

The leading causes of death today are chronic diseases, such as cardiovascular disease, diabetes, and, you guessed it, autoimmunity. Autoimmune conditions such as lupus are on the rise and are quickly becoming epidemics worldwide.

The problem is, chronic diseases are vastly different from infectious diseases. While an antibiotic can fix the problem when it comes to killing off a bad bacteria, pharmaceuticals given for treating chronic conditions such as lupus are simply Band-Aids. *If you have to take something long term for it to continue to manage the problem, is it actually fixing anything?* Unfortunately, no, and this is where the medical model is no longer viable. This is a major reason why patients in the standard model of care are not getting better and tend to get worse with time. This is why doctors expect to see their patients get worse with time and not better because that's what they see routinely. Because of this frustration, many doctors have started seeking out alternative practices to help their patients. Doctors become doctors to help people. All the time, schooling, late nights, money, blood, sweat, and tears that go into getting a doctorate are driven by a passion to help people, and many doctors have been failed by the medical model as well.

While the medical model isn't going to change overnight, you can do something about it. You can start to take control of your own health. You can start to educate yourself on how to take care of your body. And by doing this, you decide the outcome. Everyone deserves to understand how to take care of their body. A diagnosis is the opportunity to do just that. Because in order to be able to fix a problem, you first have to understand it.

CHAPTER THREE

Understanding Autoimmunity

To understand the immune system, you have to understand where it lives. Approximately 80 percent of your immune system actually lives in your gut, or gastrointestinal track. What!? Why the heck would your immune system live in your gut? Isn't your gut just meant to break down food? New research is emerging all the time looking at how the gut does so much more than just digest food. When you take a look at what is actually happening under the microscope in the intestines, it makes sense that your immune system lives there.

The gut barrier or the wall of cells that line the intestines not only has the important job of absorbing nutrients from food but is also the wall that keeps things from getting straight into the bloodstream. On the other side of that wall is the immune system. And this is genius because that is where most of our exposure to the outside world happens, and that is where your immune system is needed most to be able to combat anything that could be harmful.

We get exposed to things like bad bacteria, parasites, and viruses all the time in our food, water, and environment; therefore, it is necessary for the system in our body that protects us from those things to be the first line of defense to protect from those things getting into our bodies. Sometimes, however, it isn't the more obvious "bad guys" that trigger our immune system into overdrive. More often than not, it is what we do and what we get exposed to on a daily basis that matters most when understanding autoimmunity.

Our immune systems are innately designed to protect us. Autoimmunity by definition is an abnormal response of this very special system, but this doesn't just happen without cause. In the following chapters we will discuss in detail the common reasons why the autoimmune process happens to help you better understand the real underlying causes of autoimmunity and teach you the tools you need to fix them for good.

PART TWO

Getting to the Root Cause

CHAPTER FOUR

Main Triggers/
Root Causes of Lupus

Over the years we have seen common trends in patients with lupus and autoimmunity and have identified eight common underlying dysfunctions that can tend to lead to the overactivation of the immune system and trigger and perpetuate the disease process. The eight issues shown in the following chart all play a role in regulating the immune system and need to be evaluated for every person suffering from an autoimmune disease.

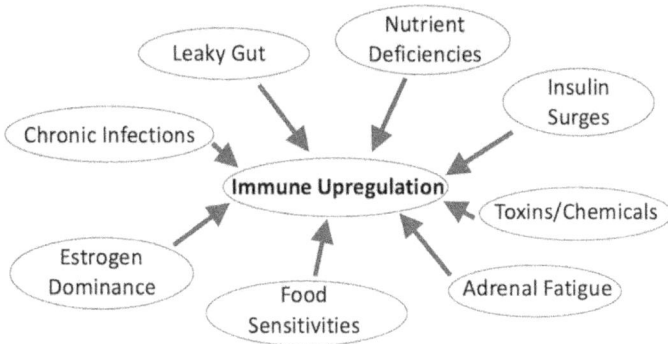

Diagram showing eight triggers pointing toward "Immune Upregulation": Leaky Gut, Nutrient Deficiencies, Insulin Surges, Chronic Infections, Toxins/Chemicals, Estrogen Dominance, Food Sensitivities, Adrenal Fatigue.

Leaky Gut

The term *leaky gut* might sound strange, but our guts are made to be "leaky" to some degree. Our gastrointestinal system, the long tube that makes up our digestive tract and leads from mouth to anus, is also a very important barrier to separate us from the outside world and what we get exposed to on a daily basis. This "tube" is made up of cells that create a wall that keeps things from getting directly into our bloodstream. Our cells are connected with tight junctions that fit together like puzzle pieces or Legos. When things like food particles are broken down into small enough particles, they can be absorbed though the cells and cell junctions to get into the bloodstream, where they can circulate to get to the cells that need them. These junctions are small enough that larger particles, things like undigested foods and bacteria, can't normally get through to get into circulation. This protects us from exposure to potentially harmful substances and only allows things in that will benefit us.

However, sometimes this important barrier can be breached, causing things like undigested food, chemicals, and bacteria to get into our bloodstream. This is called increased intestinal permeability, or "leaky gut." But remember, this gut barrier is also home to about 80 percent of our immune system, and its job is to identify foreign and potentially harmful invaders to fight them off before they can make us sick or cause harm. When we have leaky gut and too many things are getting through that barrier, it puts our immune system on high alert and cranks up our defenses. This upregulation of the immune system from leaky gut is a common underlying cause in creating an abnormal immune response in the body and a cause of autoimmunity.

Food Sensitivities

The very food you eat on a regular basis may be contributing to your symptoms and upregulating your immune system. Food sensitivities are your immune system's aberrant response to a non-harmful substance. This creates inflammation and can further perpetuate leaky gut, leading to an increased risk of developing more food reactions.

When you eat a food, let's say broccoli, it has to be broken down and digested into small nutrients for your body to be able to absorb and benefit from it. When your gut barrier is unhealthy or "leaky," undigested food particles can sometimes get through the gut wall and into the bloodstream before they are completely broken down. Since your immune system isn't normally exposed to large undigested food particles, it can easily mistake this large undigested piece of broccoli for something that isn't supposed to be there and treat it more like a bacteria than a piece of food. This mistaken identity can cause your immune system to attack the broccoli and upregulate the rest of your immune system to be on high alert to look for anything else that looks like that "harmful" piece of broccoli.

When your immune system identifies something as harmful, your body makes these "memory cells" that remember what it looks like so if you get exposed to it again, it will remember that it is bad and attack it before it can make you sick. These memory cells are called immunoglobulins or antibodies. This is how vaccines work. If you inject a virus into your bloodstream, you are causing your immune system to make these antibodies to remember how to fight off this virus if you get exposed to it in the future.

Now we know broccoli isn't bad for you, but if your immune system makes antibodies to it, every time you eat broccoli, you risk turning on your immune system and triggering inflammation and possibly an autoimmune reaction with certain foods. Now that normally healthy food can actually be causing more harm than good. This abnormal reaction to food can actually be a root cause of triggering autoimmunity. The reason for this is that certain foods, when not properly digested, look similar enough to some of your cells or tissues in your body and therefore can cause a case of mistaken identity with your immune system. For example, when your immune system is exposed to say, gluten, the protein in wheat, it looks similar enough to some of the tissues in your body such as your thyroid gland that it can cause your immune system to mistakenly attack your thyroid. This is called molecular mimicry and can be a root cause of how the food you eat can be a triggering or perpetuating factor in your autoimmunity. We will discuss how to identify these food sensitivities and what you can do about them more later.

Food also supplies us with the needed nutrients to keep our immune system functioning properly. Nutrient deficiencies can contribute to the overall inability of your immune system to keep you safe but can also play a role in causing your immune system to overreact to normal foods.

While the foods you eat could play a large role in how your immune system works, many other factors can impact a healthy immune system. In the following chapters we will discuss not only how to identify if the foods you are eating are contributing to your immune upregulation but also identify what you should be eating to avoid nutrient deficiencies that contribute to the overall immune dysfunction. Food can truly be the most powerful medicine.

Chronic Infections

When we talk about infections, most people think of symptoms like stuffy nose, sore throat, fever, nausea, etc. But infections don't always have to show up with the typical head cold or flu symptoms; in fact, some infections are more silent and chronic and don't necessarily have obvious symptoms. Different categories of chronic infections include things like viruses (Epstein-Barr that causes mono and chronic fatigue), hepatitis, and Lyme disease that live in the body and can be dormant for years without active symptoms. Then, there are also bacterial infections that change the bacteria in our guts or our microbiome; these include things like H. pylori, C. diff, and yeast infections, such as candida. Parasites can also sometimes be found in places like the gut and cause infection. A lot of these "gut infections" don't present with the typical signs like fever and nausea but rather can play an important role in upregulating the immune system in the gut and activating or perpetuating autoimmunity. Chronic infections can also wear down the immune system over time.

People with lupus tend to have higher levels of antibodies to some viruses compared to people without lupus. Some of the most common viral infections connected to lupus include Epstein-Barr virus (EBV), cytomegalovirus (CMV), parvovirus, and herpes virus. Parvovirus can actually cause symptoms very similar to lupus but will go away over time.

Dormant (asymptomatic/inactive) viruses survive in the body stored in body tissues. This is one possible reason why certain body tissues may be more attacked by the immune system than others. This could be one reason some people have certain symptoms such as arthritis if there are foreign bodies or viruses in the joint tissues.

Lab testing can show if someone has had recent or past exposure to these viruses. When the immune system is exposed to a foreign substance, such as a virus, it produces antibodies to that substance to remember it next time it encounters it. By looking at different immune markers on your blood, you can see if your immune system has recently been exposed to the foreign substance or has just had past exposure.

Nutrient Deficiencies

Perhaps one of the most important factors in controlling our health comes down to having the right ingredients. Just like you need to have the right ingredients when making a cake, our bodies need the proper ingredients to heal and be healthy. Our bodies come equipped with an innate capacity to heal. If you scrape your knee or get a paper cut, your body innately knows how to heal the wound, and eventually, it will disappear. Our bodies are very intelligent in healing but need the right tools to do so.

Nutrient deficiencies can come from simply not eating enough nutrient-rich foods, which is why proper diet is extremely important. But they can also come from poor digestion. If you are not able to digest and absorb the nutrients from your food, it doesn't matter how well you are eating. In order to have a good nutrient status, you need to not only consume the right foods but ensure that your gut is healthy and processing things appropriately.

Vitamin D is arguably the most important vitamin (also considered a pro-hormone) for immune system balance. Most people are deficient and do not get enough vitamin D from their diet or lifestyle to help support the very important role it plays when it comes to health.

Toxins and Chemicals

The average woman applies somewhere in the neighborhood of 200–500 chemicals to her body before she even walks out the door in the morning! Think about all she puts on: the shampoo, conditioner, body wash, creams and lotions, makeup, deodorant, nail polish, and hair products. It's not too hard to believe! But what effect do all these chemicals have on our bodies? They're just on our skin, right? They aren't actually getting into our bodies, are they? Wrong. Many of the chemicals we apply to our bodies actually get absorbed through our skin. This leads to a huge amount of chemical exposure to our immune system. Remember, our skin is one of our largest organs and a barrier system, just like our gut, that is meant to keep things out of our bodies, and it is a place where our immune systems are constantly surveying and protecting us from the outside world. So, what happens when we apply these chemicals to our skin? This constant exposure to a plethora of man-made substances keeps our immune systems on high alert as they try to protect us from any external dangers we encounter, including those from our daily beauty routines.

Adrenals

Let's talk about stress. Stress is potentially the most important factor when talking about health. But what is stress? Stress refers to our body's response to its environment and comes in many forms: physical (like a fall or a trauma), chemical (such as toxins, foods, excess hormones), and mental/emotional (such as things we all deal with in our daily lives—deadlines, timelines, relationships). Not all stress is bad; it is simply the way our body deals with all the things it encounters on a daily basis.

Let's say a tiger jumped out from behind you right now. A healthy stress response would be to jump up and try to run away. Stress guides our body's safety mechanisms and tells our body what to do for survival. But what if that stress we are talking about is a bee sting or a traffic jam on your way to work? Your body perceives stress as stress no matter the cause. So, whether or not you are being chased by a tiger or reacting to a food you ate, your body goes into survival mode and releases stress hormones to try to "save" you. One of the major stress hormones is cortisol, a hormone produced by the adrenal glands, the little glands that sit on top of your kidneys. If your adrenal glands are not functioning correctly, it negatively affects the immune system and a number of functions in the body that are tied to cortisol, such as your sleep/wake cycle, blood sugar control, and energy. Too much cortisol has been shown to cause leaky gut and negatively impacts conversion of other hormones. For example, too much cortisol can block the production and conversion of the thyroid hormone, the hormone that controls cell metabolism. Cortisol is also a fat-storing hormone and is commonly a cause of belly fat and weight gain.

A Word About Cortisol, the Adrenals, and Menopause

Too many women accept the belief that menopause symptoms (hot flashes, night sweats, mood swings, and vaginal dryness) are a normal part of aging and are to be expected. This is simply not true. Menopause symptoms are just that—symptoms. They are just the body's way of communicating that something is off or not working properly. These symptoms are signaling a shift in hormone production, which naturally changes around this time. However, the body does not just stop making hormones after menopause. Once the ovaries shut down their production of hormones, the adrenal glands take over. When this transition is smooth, there are no "menopause symptoms," just a normal continuation (albeit lower) of hormone production. A smooth transition into menopause requires good adrenal health. Years of chronic stress and sleep issues can cause suboptimal adrenal function and lead to a poor transition into menopause. This is one reason why it is critical to have good adrenal gland function so you can prevent or reverse dreaded menopause symptoms.

Insulin and Blood Sugar

Sometimes seemingly "simple" problems such as blood sugar issues—hypoglycemia (low blood sugar), hyperglycemia (high blood sugar), prediabetes, diabetes, and insulin resistance—can cause massive problems under the surface and cause your health to fail at a cellular level. Many times, blood sugar problems, such as insulin resistance (when your cells no longer respond to the hormone insulin to allow sugar into the cell), are at the root of dysfunction and inflammation in the body, especially in autoimmunity. Sometimes the foundations of health are broken. Like when glucose (sugar) can't get into the cell due to something like insulin resistance, your cell cannot produce ATP (cellular energy) and, therefore, can't work as efficiently. Just like your car won't go if it runs out of gas, all cell function suffers if your cells can't produce ATP. This is why one of the foundations of healthy cell function is proper blood sugar control and insulin sensitivity.

When this foundation is dysfunctional, it affects all your cells, leading to system-wide problems. One common symptom of insulin resistance is fatigue, especially after meals. Have you ever wanted to take a nap after lunch or experienced the all-too-common energy crash in the afternoon where suddenly you are reaching for that candy bar or cup of coffee to keep going? One danger with insulin resistance is that is it "silent." It is the main mechanism behind diabetes and prediabetes, and yet even people with a "normal" A1c (the marker used to test for diabetes) can have insulin resistance and not know it. It is estimated that over half the population in the US has either diabetes or prediabetes, and yet a majority of those have no idea and remain undiagnosed. The sad thing is most of the time even when someone is diagnosed with prediabetes, it is not taken seriously until it becomes diabetes. This is a problem because the only difference between diabetes and prediabetes is really just a lab value. Blood sugar problems can be reversed and no one is destined to be or become diabetic, but you have to know you have the problem to be able to solve it, and many times it is being missed.

Insulin is a hormone that gets glucose into our cells for cell energy production. However, too much of a good thing is not always a good thing, and this is especially true for insulin. Insulin is actually very inflammatory. It is also a fat-storing hormone and is often responsible for that stubborn belly fat. Due to the inflammatory nature of insulin, it is a known trigger and perpetuator of immune system upregulation. Insulin surges can happen when something called insulin resistance is present. Insulin resistance refers to the insulin receptors on the cell membranes not responding to that hormone signal (example of signal being ignored). When this happens, your pancreas, the organ that releases insulin, has to release more and more insulin to try to get the cell to respond. The cells need to respond to the insulin's signal as this allows glucose (sugar) to get into the cell from our blood and create cell energy. When you have excess insulin, it is very inflammatory and destructive in the body, and it causes your immune system to be on high alert, as if it were a foreign invader or bacteria. This is why underlying blood sugar problems can trigger autoimmunity and can make it worse.

Hormones/Estrogen Dominance

A common question that comes up with autoimmunity is, Why do most autoimmune diseases affect women more than men? While a number of factors, including genetics even down to the chromosomes, affect this, the likely answer may have to do with the hormone estrogen. Estrogen, just like insulin, is an inflammatory hormone. And even though both men and women produce estrogen, women make a lot more of it and have way more fluctuations with their hormones, especially at different times in their life. It is not uncommon to see autoimmune problems develop at times when the hormones are fluctuating the most: puberty, pregnancy, post pregnancy, menopause, and perimenopause.

Estrogen surges or estrogen dominance (an imbalance between estrogen and progesterone) can be the perfect inflammatory response to trigger your immune system to be on guard. Too much estrogen can stem from a number of reasons, such as an overproduction (from things like uterine fibroids) or poor detox and clearance of estrogen. The liver plays a major role in hormone balance with things like estrogen dominance because it is responsible for breaking down excess hormones to be excreted from the body. Poor detox pathways or genetic problems inhibit proper breakdown of excess estrogen and lead to dangerous estrogen metabolites known to increase risk of certain cancers, such as breast cancer. But detox mechanisms in the gut can also contribute to higher estrogen in the body, such as high levels of beta glucuronidase, which is a by-product of having overgrowths of bad bacteria or yeast in the gut. High levels of beta glucuronidase cause the reabsorption of toxins, such as excess estrogen, that are supposed to be eliminated in the stool to be reabsorbed back into our bodies. Making too much estrogen and not being able to clear it from our system both lead to excess estrogens, which are inflammatory and potentially harmful.

A majority of women who develop lupus do so in their childbearing years (from puberty to menopause). It is also not uncommon for symptoms of lupus to increase or worsen around their monthly cycle as the hormones fluctuate.

A Word on Genetics and Lupus

While our genetics can certainly play a role in development of autoimmunity, we also know through the study of epigenetics that changes in diet and lifestyle also play a large role in the development of autoimmune diseases. Since many of the problematic genes are found on the X chromosome and females have two while males have only one, women already have twice the risk of having gene abnormalities that lead to lupus compared to men. But we know that gene expression can be modified and risk factors minimized. Remember, just because you have genetic abnormalities or are more susceptible to developing something doesn't mean you are destined to have it. Even if the disease has already been triggered, lifestyle factors impact the disease progression and can help keep the disease inactive or in a state of remission. Genetics are just a small part of the overall picture with lupus, and fortunately, we have control over a majority of the factors that impact the disease path.

Other Causes

Medications

Certain medications have been shown to cause lupus. When a medication causes lupus, it is referred to as drug-induced lupus, and the symptoms will go away when the drug is stopped. Some of the common medications that have been shown to cause lupus include hydralazine, methyldopa, procainamide, and isoniazid. A large percentage of people with lupus also react poorly to the sulfa antibiotic Bactrim or Septra. This antibiotic has been shown to cause immune flares and allergic reactions in people with lupus. Thus, it is recommended people with lupus avoid this antibiotic.

Environmental Factors/Triggers

Sunlight exposure is a known cause/trigger and perpetuating factor in lupus. The sun's ultraviolet rays (UVA and UVB) cause chemical reactions in our skin. One of the benefits of UV light exposure is the production of vitamin D, which happens when our skin is exposed to UV light. However, certain UV rays, specifically UVA-2 and UVB rays, can cause damage to the skin cells and cause an overreaction with the immune system. Our skin is one of our biggest barriers of our body and is one such place our immune system interacts with and gets exposure to our outside environment. For people with lupus, these UV rays can upregulate the immune response and trigger autoimmunity to begin or worsen. For this reason, people with lupus need to avoid or minimize UV exposure. Another source of UV exposure comes from indoor lighting, and certain precautions need to be taken to minimize the harmful exposure to such lights in the home and/or workplace.

Chemical Exposure

Most people know the dangers of cigarette smoking in this day and age. But one of the lesser-known dangers associated with cigarette smoking is higher risk of developing lupus and other autoimmune diseases. Tobacco contains high amounts of toxic chemicals, such as hydrazine, cadmium, and insecticides.

Limiting chemical exposure is important in keeping a happy immune system, and not only is cigarette smoking highly toxic, but it also increases oxidative stress in the body, which leads to stress on the immune system.

Exposure to silica, a natural mineral, has been shown to have effects on the immune system. People in certain occupations can get too much exposure: stone, ceramic, or pottery work; highway construction; computer wafers; dry cleaning; and janitorial work.

Phthalates and solvents, toxic groups of chemicals that people can get exposed to daily in their home or occupation, can also lead to immune issues. Phthalates are synthetic chemicals found in a number of forms, such as plastics, rubber, paints, cleaners, enteric-coated pills, fabric softeners, and cosmetics. Solvents are found in products like paints, nail polish, dyes, and processing film. In order to avoid or minimize toxic exposure, use more natural plant-based alternatives.

All About Balance

When it comes to overall function in the body, it comes back to the very basic principle of homeostasis or balance. All the systems in the body work best within certain parameters, and deviation from these optimal set points leads to dysfunction. Your immune system is no different. We will discuss more about balancing the immune system later.

Nicole's Health Journey

After a thorough health history, it was apparent that multiple aspects of Nicole's daily life were contributing to her overall poor health, and further investigation with lab testing helped us quickly identify the underlying causes of her inflammation and immune upregulation.

Nicole was following the Standard American Diet, SAD diet, for short, eating many inflammatory foods and missing a lot of necessary nutrients and variety in her diet needed for health and immune function. She also had signs of poor digestion, was skipping meals frequently due to her crazy schedule, and was under a lot of stress.

Her labs showed several problems:

- High levels of inflammation

- High antibodies for lupus and Sjogren's

- Low levels of vitamin D

- White blood cell counts showing signs of infection

- Low blood sugar

- Adrenal glands not working as well as they should

- Estrogen levels showing signs of estrogen dominance

- Multiple overgrowths of bad bacteria in her gut and leaky gut (shown through a fecal stool test)

In order to get her lupus under control and regain her health, Nicole was going to have to make some changes in her diet and lifestyle. She knew it wouldn't be easy, but she finally had the answers and a plan to start taking control of her health and moving in the right direction.

CHAPTER FIVE

Food Overview

The Key to Health Is through the Gut

We grow up learning that our gut, or gastrointestinal system, is simply the system that digests our food and eliminates waste from our bodies. But our guts are so much more! What if I were to tell you that our bodies house ten times more bacteria than human cells? Yes, you read that right. A healthy gut contains about three pounds of good bacteria that make up what is called our microbiome. More and more research is looking to the gut microbiome as a connection to not only gut function but overall health and vitality. Just as we talked about earlier, this also plays a role in a healthy immune system as our guts also house about 80 percent of our immune systems! This amazing part of our body not only plays a major role in keeping us healthy but can also be one of the biggest areas of dysfunction when we are unwell.

What the Heck Do I Eat?

When it comes to the important task of answering the question, What the heck do I eat? a great place to start is a plan called the elimination diet. Since many people who experience adverse reactions to food don't realize that a specific food is causing symptoms, and because food reactions are often overlooked as a contributor to chronic health issues, the elimination diet is an excellent tool to help identify reactions to foods. The main types of reactions one can have to a food fall into three categories: allergy, intolerance, sensitivity.

An allergy is an immune reaction to a food. These reactions usually come on right away after exposure and can be severe and even life-threatening to some. Common allergy reactions are things like anaphylaxis and hives. Other symptoms could be milder, such as a swollen tongue or runny nose, but they come on immediately after exposure. Many people are already aware they have an allergy before doing an elimination diet and therefore should continue to avoid that food even if it is allowed on the diet.

When it comes to food intolerance, the most common intolerance people are aware of is lactose intolerance.

Unlike an allergy, food intolerances are not a reaction with your immune system, but rather an inability to digest that part of the food. This can be things like lacking the digestive enzymes to break down the sugar in milk (lactose intolerance) or the inability of your liver to process things like alcohol or caffeine. If your body has a hard time breaking something down, it is more likely to mistake it for being harmful. Common food intolerances include things like lectins (the part of the plant that protects itself from being digested), histamines, and preservatives, such as sulfites, and these reactions cause inflammation in the body, leading to problems like pain or overall discomfort.

Food sensitivities are a delayed immune response that can come on hours to days to a week after exposure. This can make it tricky to identify especially since symptoms tend to be less severe and not as obvious as an allergy reaction that shows up right away. Symptoms vary widely and can be anything from headaches, runny nose, joint pain, skin issues, bloating, bowel changes, fatigue, mood changes, or weight changes.

After completing the elimination diet, you can start to reintroduce foods back into your diet to test out any reactions. Staying on a restricted diet and not eating foods you no longer have to avoid isn't necessarily healthy. Most likely you will not have to continue to avoid everything eliminated long term. That's why the reintroduction phase is extremely important as you want to make sure you catch any reactions that might be there but also be able to add back foods that don't cause a reaction. As eager as you may be to add everything back in at once, it is important to add things back slowly and one at a time for the best test. To best do this, you should add back one new thing to the diet by eating it multiple times within that first day. Then you stop eating it and wait at least forty-eight hours to see if anything changes or you have a reaction.

It is always a good idea to track what you are doing by keeping a log or journal of what food you added and when you added it so you can watch for any subsequent reactions. If you suspect you had a reaction to a food, continue to keep it out of the diet for a few more months before trying to reintroduce it again. If you don't notice any reactions, you may keep that food in and add back the next food.

Foods to Avoid

Besides the typical foods eliminated during an elimination diet such as wheat and dairy, there are a few unique foods to also potentially avoid for someone with lupus. Alfalfa sprouts and mung bean sprouts both contain high levels of the amino acid L-canavanine, which has been shown to stimulate the immune system. Alfalfa sprouts specifically have been shown to be linked to the onset of SLE. People with SLE should avoid alfalfa and mung bean sprouts.

Garlic is known for its beneficial anti-inflammatory and antimicrobial properties. However, it is also thought to potentially increase activity of the immune system, and some doctors recommend avoiding garlic for those with autoimmunity even though there isn't any evidence of causing autoimmunity in humans.

Creating a Healthy Relationship with Food

We've all been there . . . Have a bad day? Feeling run down? Depressed? Stressed? Do your emotions cause you to crave or reach for certain comfort foods?

For many people, food is more than a necessity for life. Food is commonly associated with comfort, pleasure, joy, social engagement, community, and reward.

People commonly think, "I've been eating well all week, I think I will **treat myself** to some ice cream." While this way of thinking of food as a reward or treat may seem benign, viewing your food this way may be holding you back from getting better. Just think about the top foods you "reward" yourself with or use as comfort. Broccoli probably isn't what came to mind. Usually the things we "treat" ourselves with are things we know are not good for us, hence why we save them for a special occasion or reason. Whether or not you are feeling good or feeling bad, using sugar-laden or inflammatory foods is *not* a way to reward your body; *it is sabotage!* Would you be treating yourself with a little bowl of rat poison? Hopefully not! Then why would you reward yourself with something that you know is not good for you and harms your health?

Challenge: Next time you want to "treat" yourself, choose something that isn't food related. How about something like a massage or spa day? Try out a new gym class or exercise. Go to a new museum with a friend. Do something that makes you laugh. Do something that will help heal your body, not harm it.

Using Nutrients as Tools

Just as a carpenter needs a hammer or a seamstress needs thread, our bodies need tools to heal and repair and work optimally: nutrients!

In today's day and age, it is nearly impossible to get all you need from food because our food isn't as healthy as it once was and does not supply all the nutrients we need, especially when the body is under stress or inflamed. This is why nutraceutical support can be essential for helping the body heal, and by knowing what specific issues need to be addressed, you can supplement appropriately.

Diet and lifestyle play major roles in determining our overall health, but sometimes they are not sufficient for supplying all the necessary "ingredients" for healing, especially when the body is under stress or inflamed. Using added nutrients to *supplement* our healthy habits can be a game changer in terms of speed of healing. Our bodies are intelligent and very capable of healing and adapting; however, by the time someone develops symptoms or is diagnosed with a condition or disease, our bodies have usually already been trying to adapt and compensate for some time, and our resources are worn out. Replenishing those resources through supplementation can be an important step in giving the body what it needs for the healing process.

Remember, you aren't just what you eat, you are what you digest and absorb.

Supplement vs. Nutraceutical

A supplement is a product taken orally that contains one or more ingredients (such as vitamins or amino acids) that are intended to supplement one's diet and are not considered food. Nutraceuticals are pharmaceutical-grade supplements that contain synergistic blends of vitamins, minerals, and/or herbs with a specific purpose of assisting in treating a specific disease process or physiologic dysfunction. Supplements are widely available for purchase over the counter, whereas nutraceuticals are recommended or prescribed by healthcare providers. Nutraceuticals are best used when addressing underlying root problems as they assist in the body's natural innate healing process and can aid in quicker recovery. It is recommended that you seek the help of a trained professional for assistance in supplementation.

A Word on Quality

Quality matters when it comes to safety and effectiveness with supplementation. While many of the recommended nutrients can be found over the counter at most health food stores, it is wise to use caution when buying these products as many times the cheaper form of nutrients used are not very absorbable in the body and, therefore, not as effective.

Form matters as well. Vitamin D, for example, is better absorbed as a liquid tincture under the tongue. This way of dosing also allows for higher amounts to be taken and absorbed for optimal benefit.

Foundational Nutrients

Certain key nutrients are needed across the board for general health and well-being. Additional nutrients can help support the body at times of need and can be a catalyst for healing and knocking down inflammation. Here are a few key nutrients needed for a good foundation:

- **Vitamin D3**: Vitamin D3 is perhaps one of the most important vitamins and essential for regulating the immune system. Most people are deficient in this important nutrient.

- **B Vitamins**: B vitamins are at the core of foundational cell functions and impact everything from energy to brain function and your ability to detox.

- **Healthy fats/omegas**: Omegas, especially the anti-inflammatory omega 3s, play a role in healing, decreasing inflammation, and supporting the immune system.

- **Multivitamins**: A good multivitamin can help fill in the gaps of an already healthy diet or assist in support for someone struggling with their health.

CHAPTER SIX

Lifestyle Overview

Mental and Emotional Health

Depression is a common accompaniment with chronic health conditions, especially autoimmunity and lupus, for a number of reasons. For one, the diagnosis of a lifelong condition can be devastating. Little hope is given with lupus due to being seen and labeled as a chronic progressive degenerative disease that is expected to get worse with time, not better. And many patients look to their doctors for hope only to find disappointment when their only solution is a path of medication after medication riddled with side effects and complications.

Depression is a symptom. Just like pain, inflammation, and fatigue, depression is a way your body is trying to tell you that something isn't right. One of the biggest issues leading to depression and anxiety goes back to our gut. Our guts actually produce most of our neurotransmitters, or brain chemicals, like serotonin, that make us feel good. In order to make those feel-good brain chemicals, our guts need the right building blocks: the right nutrients and, get this, good bacteria! Again, the microbiome plays a critical role in determining our health and in this case our mental health. With a poor gut environment, not only do we not absorb nutrients and get the benefits, but we also don't feed the good bacteria in our guts, which creates imbalances with our microbiome. By eating a wide variety of plant foods in our diet and by minimizing stress in our lifestyle, we help create a good foundation for a healthy microbiome.

Many people with autoimmunity deal with emotional stress stemming from their own health struggles. Being told you have a lifelong and life-threatening disease is something no one wants to be told, but then to make things harder, most people haven't walked in their shoes and don't fully understand what they are going through or the challenges they face on a daily basis. This continual stress impacts your emotional health and physical health. We've already discussed how stress isn't bad, but it becomes a bad thing when it is chronic. When that stress doesn't go away after the threat is gone, those stress hormones that can save your life can also wreak havoc on it. We know that excess cortisol can cause issues. Too much stress is bad. But we also can't avoid all the stress in life, so how do we protect ourselves from it?

Stress management can be a powerful tool to help you learn how to not only deal with the stress in your life but also protect your body from the harmful effects of excess stress. But first you need to be able to identify what stresses your body is dealing with. What are your sources of stress, and which ones do you actually have control over? Which ones do you not? By simply identifying which stresses you have control over, you can start to make changes in your daily life to combat those, and for the stresses that are out of your control, you can practice stress management techniques to help your body cope and to negate the negative impact they have on your body. We will discuss how to identify stress and finding stress management techniques you can do in more detail later.

Healing through Breathing

Our autonomic nervous systems are composed of sympathetic and parasympathetic. The sympathetic system is commonly known as the "fight-or-flight" nervous system, and the parasympathetic system is known as "rest and digest." Both of these systems play a role in keeping us alive on a daily basis without us even being conscious of it. The sympathetic nervous system controls functions such as keeping your heart beating and keeping you breathing, while the parasympathetic system controls functions such as gut motility and restorative sleep. When our bodies are under stress, we are in a more sympathetic dominant state.

See the resources at the end of this book for a simple breathing exercise you can start doing today to manage stress and promote healing.

A Health Buddy

Whether it's a shoulder to cry on, an ear to listen, someone to understand, or someone to keep you accountable, we all need help and support sometimes. Finding a "health buddy" or someone you can connect with to help you along the way can make a huge difference in ease and success. If you don't have a loved one or friend to lean on or are looking for additional support, you can find support groups online and around the country for people with lupus. Connecting with other people who are experiencing similar challenges with their health can be very healing in itself. Human connection, understanding, and empathy play a major role in the mental, emotional, and spiritual aspect of healing.

Tip: Join groups of people who are optimistic and surround yourself with people who inspire you to be better. Learn from those who have done what you want to do. Avoid negativity and don't be afraid to walk away from toxic people. Negativity, including negative self-talk, only holds you back from achieving your goals, whatever they may be. Having a supporting team to back you up only makes you stronger.

PART THREE

Tools and Therapies

A Deeper Dive into Implementing Changes

As you will notice in the following chapters, there are no specific "protocols" for joint pain or headaches or fatigue, since as we discussed earlier, symptoms are just indicators, not the actual problem. The following recommendations are generalized support for some of the most common underlying issues in autoimmunity. We encourage you to work with a certified functional medicine practitioner for more personalized recommendations and support with implementing changes. You can also check out our online resources and course by visiting caplanhealthinstitute.com.

We will be diving into each of the main areas that commonly need to be addressed as they relate to lupus and autoimmunity as a whole. We will take a look and highlight simple changes you can start to implement as they relate to food and nutrition, lifestyle, and nutrient therapy to start to move toward your health goals.

CHAPTER SEVEN

Insulin and Blood Sugar

Food and Nutrition for Healthy Blood Sugar

When it comes to stabilizing blood sugar or reversing insulin resistance, *what's on the end of your fork* can be one of the most powerful tools you have. When it comes to eating healthy, a lot of people think that just means eliminating fat. Not all fat is equal. If you are not eating fat to avoid weight gain, you may be doing more harm than good. Incorporating good healthy fats into your diet is essential in overall health, not to mention hormone regulation. Adding healthy fats such as olive oil, avocado, coconut, and nuts and seeds into your diet can be helpful in keeping you full and satisfied and keeping your blood sugar stable between meals.

Following a low-glycemic food plan, such as a modified version of the Mediterranean diet, paleo diet, or low-carb ketogenic diet, can be helpful guides to navigate what to eat.

The key things to emphasize when it comes to blood sugar stabilizing the effects of foods are low glycemic, low carbohydrate, and high fiber.

Blood Sugar Specific	
Eat	**Avoid**
Whole, fresh, local, seasonal foods (grass-fed, wild, organic animal proteins, and produce)	Foods with added sugar (includes sugar, sugar substitutes, sucrose and fructose, and sugar-sweetened beverages)
Healthy fats like extra virgin olive oil, olives, avocado oil, almonds, cashews, hazelnuts, macadamia nuts, pecans, flax seeds	Refined and/or processed carbohydrates (includes carbohydrates from refined starches (e.g., white-flour breads and pasta)
Green tea	Trans fats
Mixed nuts	Overly cooked foods/ charred foods/ fried foods
Cinnamon	Fruit juices
High omega-3 fatty fish	Large meals
Low-glycemic vegetables	
Adequate hydration (divide body weight in pounds by 2 to get daily recommended water intake in ounces (e.g., a person weighing 150 pounds should consume at least 75 ounces of water daily)	

Lifestyle for Healthy Blood Sugar

How and *when* we eat, and our other important and sometimes easily overlooked lifestyle habits, are just as important as *what* we eat in terms of impacting our blood sugar.

Let's talk about timing of meals. First, you need to determine if you tend to get high blood sugars or low blood sugars.

Symptoms of low blood sugar, or **hypo***glycemia*, include getting sweaty; feeling shaky, dizzy, or lightheaded; having a fast heart rate; feeling hungry (*or hangry*); and getting more energy after eating.

High blood sugar, or **hyper***glycemia*, can present as getting blurry vision, feeling weak, feeling tired especially after meals, and feeling an increased need to drink and urinate.

People who tend to have higher blood sugars tend to benefit most from skipping snacks and incorporating intermittent fasting. People who tend to get "hangry" or get low blood sugars tend to do better when eating more consistently throughout the day. Typically snacking every three hours or so throughout the day helps keep the blood sugar from dropping and causing a rebound effect called reactive hypoglycemia, or in other words, a spike in blood sugar if the sugar drops too low. Think of it as a built-in safety mechanism to keep us out of hypoglycemia, which could be dangerous if our sugar levels drop too low. Eating consistently throughout the day by incorporating small snacks between meals can help keep blood sugar stable, therefore avoiding the problems that come from hypoglycemia and blood sugar dysregulation.

Sleep and Blood Sugar

Adequate sleep in terms of duration and quality matters greatly in terms of blood sugar stability. This is partly due to the direct connection of blood sugar and your stress hormone cortisol. Because blood sugar fluctuations are a stress in the body, cortisol is called on in times when the sugar drops or spikes too high, making cortisol a big player in blood sugar regulation. Cortisol also plays a major role in our circadian rhythms, or sleep/wake cycle. One of the functions of cortisol is stabilizing blood sugar while in the fasting state as in when you are asleep.

Problems with sleep, such as issues falling back to sleep if you wake in the middle of the night or early morning, can sometimes be a direct result of blood sugar dysfunction and cortisol surges. Therefore, not only can issues with sleep reflect possible blood sugar issues, but by fixing underlying blood sugar issues, you can fix your sleep. Not only does blood sugar affect sleep, but sleep directly affects blood sugar. It has been shown that lack of sleep increases blood sugar! It's a vicious cycle!

If you tend to get low blood sugars, sometimes a low-glycemic snack before bed, such as unsweetened plantain chips or a handful of nuts, can help keep your blood sugar more stable as you sleep to prevent blood sugar drops. If you tend to wake up in the middle of the night and have a hard time falling back to sleep, you can simply keep a handful of grapes on your nightstand and eat them upon waking, which can help you go back to sleep quicker.

To promote better sleep, you should go to bed at the same time every night and wake up at the same time every morning. This simple routine can drastically help your cortisol and blood sugar levels stay more consistent.

Exercise and Movement

Avoiding a sedentary lifestyle is an important key to blood sugar stability. Making a commitment to exercise consistently, at least four days a week, not only improves blood sugar control but can also help with stress management and cardiovascular health.

Find your level of exercise tolerance and keep a journal of type of exercise, time, intensity, and how you felt. Whether or not you enjoy weight training, cardio, high-intensity interval training, or something a little slower such as yoga or tai chi, find what gets you up and moving and make it a habit!

Nutrient Therapy for Healthy Blood Sugar

When it comes to addressing insulin resistance and blood sugar dysregulation, a number of nutrients can aid a healthy diet and lifestyle to specifically address proper blood sugar utilization.

The following list of nutrients help with blood sugar stability and insulin receptor sensitivity, which is key in reversing insulin resistance and diabetes. A number of nutraceuticals are made up of synergistic blends of these nutrients that target insulin resistance.

Nutrient/Supplementation for Blood Sugar
Berberine
Alpha-lipoic acid
Chromium
Cinnamon
Magnesium glycinate
Vanadium

CHAPTER EIGHT

Adrenals and Cortisol

Clean Eating for Adrenal Health

Eating a clean, whole foods diet free from processed or refined carbs and stimulants is helpful in maintaining proper adrenal function and stabilizing cortisol levels. If you tend to have blood sugar issues, either high blood sugars or low blood sugars, following the principles for stabilizing blood sugar will also aid in cortisol and adrenal support.

Stimulants, such as sugar and caffeine, negatively impact the adrenals by causing them to increase their cortisol output. Caffeine adds stress on the body. And for adrenals that are already overworked and/or underperforming, that added stress may not be handled well and may contribute to the adrenal dysfunction and other health issues the person is facing.

Food triggers are a very common and sometimes overlooked contributing factor to our stress load. For this reason, following an elimination diet to identify and address food reactions is an important tool and the first step to minimizing overall stress in the body. While what's on the end of your fork is important and can help remove some of the stress on the body, when it comes to overall adrenal health, how you do what you do on a regular basis matters most. Because no matter how much we try to avoid stress, life is always going to happen, and one of the best defenses is the ability to adapt.

Pay Attention to Your Body

In part due to our nature as humans and our survival instincts, we tend to notice more when things are wrong versus when things are going well. People don't usually pay attention to how often they have bowel movements until they are constipated or have to run to the bathroom with diarrhea. Being more aware of your body and listening to when things change is an important part in healing and learning. So the first step is to pay attention to your body.

Along with paying attention to signs from your body, you also need to identify your sources of stress. Daily stress is often overlooked, yet identifying where that stress is coming from and having the tools and knowledge to better avoid or control it is a key component of controlling cortisol and keeping your adrenals happy and healthy.

Exercise: When do you feel stress? Keep a journal or take note of when you feel the effects of more stress. Whether or not it is at work or home or with certain activities, by noting what you are doing or what is going on around you when you notice more symptoms or feel more stress in your body, you can track and identify what things tend to trigger more stress in your body so you can then address or avoid them.

Turning Off "Fight or Flight"

Have you ever felt that it is "too easy" to get stressed out, with every little thing triggering feelings of stress and/or anxiety? This can be partly in thanks to your autonomic nervous system. Your autonomic nervous system can be separated into sympathetic and parasympathetic. You can imagine your autonomic nervous system like a car. The sympathetic nervous system is like the gas and the parasympathetic nervous system is the brakes. In order for the car to function optimally, you need both the gas and brakes to work when needed. Now let's say you are experiencing stress, like being chased by a tiger. Your sympathetic nervous system is what controls your "fight-or-flight" response and will "turn on" to help you run away as a means of survival. When your body is under stress, this automatic response is triggered to help you either fight or flee for safety. After the stressor is gone (you outran the tiger), your body no longer needs to be in fight-or-flight mode and should be able to switch gears into a more parasympathetic state for "rest and digest." Parasympathetic state is when the body is in rest and can heal and repair.

Sometimes when the body is under chronic stress, like in an autoimmune state, that acute stress state of fight or flight doesn't turn off, and the body stays in a state of sympathetic dominance. In this sympathetic-dominant state, the body is constantly prepared and on edge for an attack or to flee. It's like being ready for a battle 24/7.

Imagine a cup full to the brim of water. Now imagine adding just a couple of drops of water and seeing the cup overflow. When the body is constantly in a more heightened sympathetic state, your stress level is constantly full to the brim and any little added stress can set it off and cause your cup to overflow. People who are caught in sympathetic dominance experience symptoms related to being in a constant stress state. If you have ever run a marathon or done intensive exercise, you know how your body feels in the days after. You may be tired, weak, sore, and achy. While all those symptoms may be normal after an acute stress, is isn't normal to feel that constantly. Imagine if your body thought it was constantly ready to run a marathon on a minute's notice. Now even daily stresses, like running late for work or getting stuck in traffic, can trigger this stress response to be heightened and affect how you feel.

Stress is a catabolic activity, meaning it breaks down tissues in the body for fuel. This constant catabolic state in itself is a constant stress contributing to that already full cup. Unfortunately, we are hardwired to be more sympathetic as a built-in survival mechanism, and we sometimes have to teach our body to switch gears. For people experiencing stress, which is pretty much everyone, learning how to control this and keep it from controlling you is key.

One of the simplest and most effective tools for controlling this stress response and switching from sympathetic to parasympathetic is how you breathe.

Exercises for Parasympathetic Stimulation

4-7-8 Breathing

- Close your mouth and inhale quietly through your nose to a mental count of **four**.

- Hold your breath for a count of **seven**.

- Exhale completely through your mouth, making a whoosh sound to a count of **eight**.

This is one breath. Now inhale again and repeat the cycle three or more times until you start to feel a little more relaxed. You may also notice your heart rate slowing down. This is also a great tool for anxiety. Doing this exercise when you first start to notice anxiety can help stop it in its tracks and prevent an anxiety attack.

Gargling

- Gargle with water intensely twice a day.

- You will know when you have gargled long enough when your eyes start watering.

This stimulates your vagus nerve, the largest parasympathetic nerve in the body to activate your rest-and-digest system, which aids in proper stress control and gastrointestinal function. People with digestive issues can also benefit from parasympathetic stimulation exercises due to the effects of the parasympathetic on bowel motility, or peristalsis.

Exercise and Sleep

You need to develop good sleep habits, which means more than just not watching TV in bed. Because timing is key when addressing the adrenals, it is important to keep consistent sleep and wake times. Timing your exercise can also play an important role in helping your adrenals work more optimally.

By incorporating a simple five-to-ten-minute high-intensity-interval workout to your morning routine, you can help support your adrenals and what's called the cortisol awakening response. The cortisol awakening response is what helps wake you up and gets your energy going for the rest of the day. This also helps for those who struggle to get out of bed in the morning. It's like fuel in your engine: *Do you want to run on a full tank or an empty one?* By getting your heart rate up first thing in the morning, you help proper cortisol production, and therefore, a proper cortisol awakening response.

While timing of exercise is important, the amount of exercise is also something to take into account. Exercise increases endorphins, improves mood, reduces anxiety, and improves sleep. But too much of a good thing isn't necessarily better. Exercise is also a catabolic activity. So adding more stress to an already stressed-out state isn't necessarily helpful and could potentially make you worse.

A good rule of thumb is, *do it, but don't overdo it.* You just need to find your exercise "tolerance." If you feel worse after exercise (beyond normal exhaustion, physical pain besides normal soreness, or a longer than typical recovery period), then you may be doing too much. While it is okay to feel tired or sore after a workout, you shouldn't be recovering in bed for the next couple of days. To find your level of exercise tolerance, simply cut back on the intensity and duration or frequency of your workouts. Instead of working out an hour a day, try twenty to thirty minutes four to five times per week. It is important that you are feeling good with the amount and type of activity you are doing.

Restorative "Me Time"

While our daily lives can sometimes be demanding, you need to make time for the one thing that matters most: *you guessed it,* yourself! Take some time, daily, weekly, monthly, to get to know your body and appreciate all it does for you. Sometimes we get so caught up in all the negatives that come along with dealing with our health issues that we don't appreciate all the positives in our life and health. When's the last time you had to tell your heart to beat or lungs to breathe? Every day we wake up, we should appreciate what our amazing bodies do for us, especially when we are not feeling well.

Incorporating some restorative practices on a regular basis can have a profound impact on our relationship with our health, especially when it comes to managing stress. Below are some ideas of things you can start doing on a regular basis for better adrenal and overall health. It is recommended you commit to practicing these things on a regular, daily basis to begin creating good habits and make it easier to do when you need it.

Restorative "Me Time" Activities

Here are a few simple things you can do to better manage stress and take some much-needed "me time." Check off the practices you already use or mark the ones you want to try!

_____ **Practice mindfulness**

_____ **Breathing techniques such as 4-7-8**

_____ **Listen to music**

_____ **Participate in social activities, visit a friend**

_____ **Laughter** *(the best medicine!)*

_____ **Guided imagery**

_____ **Meditation**

_____ **Aromatherapy**

_____ **Gratitude journal (take an inventory of all the good things in your life)**

_____ **Physical, mental, and emotional rest**

_____ **Limit electronic device use**

_____ **Epson salt bath**

_____ **Get a massage, acupuncture, or chiropractic**

Nutrient Therapy for Healthy Adrenals

So, if we can't avoid stress in life, the best we can do is adapt! That's why some of the most powerful tools for adrenal health are called adaptogens, substances that help modulate the stress response in the body. Adaptogenic herbs are known to be restorative to the adrenals. Just like the name suggests, they help the body adapt to the demand for stress hormones, especially cortisol.

Other important nutrients needed for proper adrenal function are B vitamins (B1, B5, B6, biotin, and folate), vitamin C, vitamin D, magnesium, zinc, omega-3s, and tyrosine. See the following table for a list of adaptogenic herbs and recommended nutrient support for your adrenals.

Nutrient/Supplementation for Adrenals
Adaptogenic herbs (ashwagandha, gotu kola, licorice, panax ginseng, holy basil, eleuthero, astragalus, cordyceps, reishi, rhodiola, schisandra, tulsi, maca, moringa and shilajit)
B complex (B1, B5, B6, Biotin, Folate)
Vitamin C
Magnesium
Zinc
Omega-3
Vitamin D
Tyrosine

CHAPTER NINE

Toxins and Chemicals

Minimizing Toxic Exposure from Food

When it comes to toxic exposures from food, it's not just *what* you are eating that matters but also *how* it is handled and prepared. How you prepare food can turn a healthy thing into a health hazard. Three main areas to consider are the foods themselves, the food packaging, and the food preparation.

Tips:

- Choose foods that are organically grown when possible. Say no to GMOs. Avoid adding synthetic dyes or additives.

- Avoid plastic casing, aluminum or metal cans, cellophane, and foil. When food and drinks are exposed to things like plastic or aluminum, they have the chance to leach those harmful chemicals into the food or drink and get a free ride into your body.

- Avoid fried foods and overcooked/charred foods, choose water (steaming) over frying in oil, and choose non-toxic cookware.

Yes, you read that right. It isn't just fried foods that are a problem; overcooked foods are too. How we prepare our food is just as important as what food we eat.

So what matters most when we cook? The three basic factors include time, temperature, and cookware. As a general rule of thumb, slow, low, and moist is the healthiest way to cook.

Time

Slow cooking as in a slow cooker (or a little faster in an instant pot) is a great, non-toxic way to maintain nutrients while minimizing lectins and avoiding AGEs (advanced glycation end products). AGEs are formed when foods are charred or overbrowned. Think of AGEs as basically rusting that happens when the natural sugars in the food are overcooked. Now picture that happening in your own body . . . ew! Avoiding overcooked or blackened foods will minimize these toxic end products.

Temperature

Cooking at lower temperatures also helps avoid unwanted toxins by minimizing AGEs and trans-fats and preserving the nutrients in the food. Lightly steaming vegetables helps activate the natural enzymes and preserves the phytonutrients like sulforaphane, which gives the antioxidant boost from our plant foods.

A word of caution when cooking with oils. Some oils withstand temperature better than others at what's called their "smoke point." Cooking with oil at a higher temperature can cause the oil to lose its health benefits or be converted into a more toxic form. That's why it is generally recommended that if cooking with a fat or oil, you choose one that has a higher smoke point or one that contains more saturated fat, such as coconut oil or ghee. Save the olive oil for drizzling on food after cooking for the most health benefits.

Cookware

While nonstick cookware may make things a little easier in the kitchen, the coating used to make it nonstick is toxic. Choosing healthier cookware such as ceramic or cast iron will help you avoid cooking chemicals into your food. Also pay attention to the utensils used when cooking. Stick to metal or bamboo tools to prepare the food and avoid using plastics, especially when cooking over heat is involved.

Avoiding Toxins in the Diet	
Choose	**Avoid**
Organic, non-GMO foods and beverages	GMOs and foods sprayed with herbicides
Grass-fed, lean meats and wild-caught, low-mercury fish	Crops most affected by glyphosate: soy, corn, wheat, potatoes, canola, sugar beets, cotton
Expeller-pressed, unrefined oils	Foods with added hormones or antibiotics
Filtered water (get tested for contaminants)	Foods packaged in plastic or aluminum (foil)
Whole foods vs. processed	Alcohol, caffeine, unhealthy fats, sugar, dyes, additives and artificial sweeteners
Food and drinks in glass when available (especially for storage of leftovers)	
Foods cooked slow and at low temperature	
Non-toxic cookware	

Foods That Help with Detoxing

Avoiding toxins and chemicals in our diet is a great way to overall minimize our toxic burden. But life isn't perfect and no matter how hard we may try, we are constantly exposed to polluted food, water, air, and entertainment. So how do we help our body's natural detox processes to better get those bad things out? Well, by simply adding more good foods into our diet, we can give our bodies the necessary ingredients to detox.

A number of plant foods have their own natural detox support components:

- Algaes (chlorella and spirulina): Contain protein and vitamins and are great detoxing agents as they help bind to and eliminate metals from the body.

- Turmeric: An anti-inflammatory and an antioxidant that aids in detoxification by impacting gallbladder function, therefore supporting the bile production needed for detoxification.

- Ginger: An anti-inflammatory and an antioxidant that aids in detoxification by acting as a stimulant for the digestive tract and helping bowel function and circulation to move out of the body.

- Dark leafy greens: Full of phytonutrients and fiber, which helps the bowel eliminate waste in the bowels.

- Apples: Great source of fiber and also high in malic acid, which helps cleanse the blood.

- Cruciferous vegetables (broccoli, cabbage, bok choy, and brussels sprouts): Full of sulforaphane, a chemical known for its stimulation enzymes involved in detoxification processes as well as its antioxidant effects.

Aim for nine to thirteen servings of plant foods in your diet daily, including cruciferous vegetables and fiber-rich foods to help support the body's natural detox pathways.

Creating a Hypoallergenic Home

Have you ever noticed that some of your health problems seem to go away or lessen when you are on vacation or out of town for a bit?

That might be because there are hidden sources of toxins and allergens around us all the time, *especially in our homes*. Indoor air has been shown to be up to ten times more polluted than outdoor air, and a lot of it has to do with what we are using indoors. In fact, one of the most toxic things that many of us have and use in our homes is a dishwasher! The fumes that come from washing plastics in the dishwasher are toxic, and we then breathe them in. But what about other sometimes invisible sources of toxins or allergens, such as mold and dust mites? How do we protect ourselves from these invisible dangers?

Tips:

- Properly test your environment. If you believe you may have a mold or bacteria problem in your home, you can purchase a home test kit or hire professionals to inspect and treat any problem areas.

- Control indoor humidity. Mold loves moisture. Make sure places such as the bathroom and kitchen have good circulation or leave windows open when possible to prevent mold growth.

- Minimize animal allergens. For many of us, our pets are part of the family and share the same living space (couch, beds, etc.). If someone in your household is allergic to pet dander, it is best to avoid letting the pet into their bedroom. It is also recommended to consistently dust, vacuum, and wash bedding or linens to remove pet dander and purchase a HEPA air filter to minimize allergens in the air.

- Use filters. Air and water filters can help minimize toxic exposure by removing pollutants in the water we drink and the air we breathe. A simple countertop water filter can turn tap water into bottle-quality water without the harmful microplastics found in such bottles. Air filters can be installed in air ducts and vents or stand-alone HEPA filters can be used throughout the house.

Habits That Help You Detox

Exercise is a great way to detox. Exercise improves circulation, creating better nutrient and oxygen distribution, and physically helps the body flush toxic junk out. Simply walking stimulates movement in the body, helping lymphatic drainage, gut motility, and sweating! Sweating can also be achieved through use of infrared or dry saunas and steam rooms.

Another major source of toxins is in our everyday personal care products. Even things like most toothpastes contain a multitude of chemicals that could be harmful. Think about your daily routine: lotions, moisturizers, shampoo, conditioner, makeup, hair products, etc. How many chemicals are you putting on your body every day? And yes, it matters what you put on your body, because those chemicals have the chance to be absorbed by our skin, and we can also inhale those chemical fragrances, resulting in immune reactions to them on our skin or in our respiratory system.

Look for products that have minimal ingredients as well as ingredients that are easily identifiable. For example, try switching to castile soap such as Dr. Bronner's. With minimal ingredients, it is not only safe but also multipurpose. Castile soap can replace a number of household and personal care products, such as body wash, dog shampoo, fruit rinse, dishwashing liquid, toilet scrubber as well as acting as an all-purpose cleaner!

Visit the Environmental Working Group's website at www.ewg.org for more tips and safety ratings of a number of common products. It's a great resource for learning more about your environment and how to minimize toxic exposures in everyday life.

One more area to address when it comes to toxic exposure is right in your mouth. If you have had any dental work done, such as mercury amalgams, crowns, alloy implants, and orthodontic appliances, these too can be a source of exposure.

Find a biologic dentist. Biologic dentists are trained in safe removal practices of mercury amalgams, etc., but if removal isn't an option, avoiding things such as chemical teeth-whitening agents and grinding your teeth can help minimize the release of these toxic substances into your body.

**Lifestyle Tips for Minimizing
Toxic Exposure at Home**

Avoid chemicals in personal care products
such as lotions, moisturizers, shampoo,
conditioners, makeup, sunscreen, etc.
Avoid inhalants and environmental toxicants such
as air fresheners, scented laundry detergent, fabric
softeners, candles, household cleaners, etc.

Avoid toxins from mold, dander, dust mites
Avoid smoke and other pollutants by
using air and water purifiers

Nutrient Therapy for Detoxification Support

It's simple: give the body the tools it needs, and it can do its job.
That's especially true when it comes to detoxification. Adequate
nutrients from our diet can help support the detox pathways
while lack of sufficient nutrients can hinder the ability to remove
waste and other toxic compounds from our systems.

Nutrient Support for Detoxification
Foods for Detox
Cruciferous vegetables such as broccoli, cabbage, arugula, radishes Dark leafy greens such as collard greens, kale, bok choy, chard, cilantro and parsley Sulfur-containing foods such as garlic, onion, and leeks Foods specific for liver and kidney support such as artichokes, asparagus, beets, celery, and sprouts
Herbs for Detox
Look for teas and supplements containing the following herbs
Dandelion root Milk thistle Burdock Red clover Neem

CHAPTER TEN

Hormone Balance

Food and Nutrition for Hormone Balance

When it comes to supporting hormones through food, it's important to consider all the dietary factors that impact our hormones. From blood sugar dysfunction to poor detox ability, you want to clearly identify where the hormone imbalance or issue is stemming from to best support and restore proper balance and function.

As a general rule, you want to support the body through nutrient-rich, chemical-free, unprocessed whole foods with a focus on plant foods containing fiber and phytonutrients. You want to limit or avoid caffeine, refined carbohydrates, sugar, and alcohol. You also want to be aware of and avoid xenoestrogens and chemicals in food including pesticides, herbicides, plasticizers, hormones, and antibiotics. Choose as much organic, grass-fed, wild, and simply un-messed-with foods as possible, and drink plenty of clean filtered water.

Fiber is particularly important as it not only helps create a healthy microbiome but also helps phase 3 detoxification by removing waste from the bowels. Some of the best sources of fiber are found in plant foods we eat, or *should be eating*, on a regular basis, such as broccoli, carrots, apples, beets, and other dark colorful fruits and veggies. Legumes such as beans and lentils are also high in fiber, as are nuts and seeds. A smoothie made with low-glycemic fruits and veggies can be a great way to add more fiber into your diet. You can also add in some other beneficial ingredients such as flax seed or psyllium husk.

Seed Cycling for Hormone Cycle Regulation

Seed cycling is a gentle way to help support a woman's natural hormone changes throughout the month. The first half of the menstrual cycle is called the follicular phase.

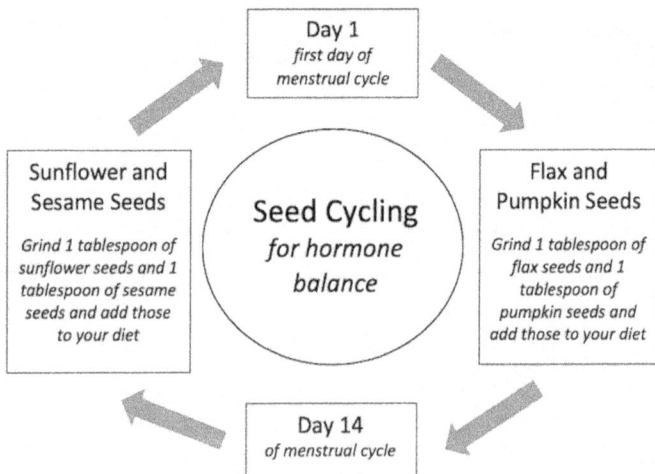

Day 1
first day of menstrual cycle

Sunflower and Sesame Seeds

Grind 1 tablespoon of sunflower seeds and 1 tablespoon of sesame seeds and add those to your diet

Seed Cycling *for hormone balance*

Flax and Pumpkin Seeds

Grind 1 tablespoon of flax seeds and 1 tablespoon of pumpkin seeds and add those to your diet

Day 14
of menstrual cycle

Consuming flax and pumpkin seeds in the follicular phase may help in a couple of ways:

1. Binding to and helping eliminate excess estrogen

2. Preventing excess testosterone and preparing the body to produce progesterone in the luteal phase from the high amounts of zinc found in pumpkin seeds

Consuming sunflower and sesame seeds during the second half of the monthly cycle, or what's called the luteal phase, can help with:

1. Progesterone production, which is peak during the luteal phase

2. Maintaining the balance between estrogen and progesterone since these seeds are high in essential fatty acids

In general, consuming a healthy diet full of nutrient-dense plant foods as well as addressing any other contributing underlying health issues is the key to regaining and maintaining hormone balance.

Eating at the Right Time

One of the biggest modifiable lifestyle issues we find contributing to hormonal imbalance has to do with when we eat.

Many people with underlying hormonal imbalances will experience weight gain as a symptom. Weight gain, the inability to lose weight, or being unable to maintain a normal weight is a sign that your hormones are to blame. That is partly because some hormones act to store fat, while others act to burn fat, and an imbalance that favors fat-storing hormones suddenly makes losing or maintaining weight very challenging if not impossible.

So, when you look up "how to lose weight" and everything tells you to "just eat less," less calories, less carbs, less sugar, less fat, etc., too many people think that just means "less" is better. But all too often we see people trying to lose weight the wrong way, by not eating regularly and at the right times. This causes issues with your hormones and actually could be a contributing factor to not being able to lose weight.

1. Not eating when it is time to eat can create blood sugar dysfunction for someone who tends to get hypoglycemic. *Remember when we were talking about low blood sugar being just as much of an issue as high blood sugar?* Well, if you are someone who tends to get "hangry," not eating when you should may not be the best approach for you. If your blood sugar is not stable, every time it drops the body has to correct it, and it tends to overcorrect it, leading to a subsequent spike in sugar, which then creates a need for more insulin. The drop in blood sugar stimulates the release of two fat-storing hormones: cortisol and insulin. So, if you tend to get low blood sugar, not eating can make you gain weight.

2. Eating erratically or skipping meals can lead to your body not knowing when the next meal is coming. This can actually cause your body to revert to its safety mechanism back from our ancestors' hunter-gatherer days when they didn't know when their next meal was. This erratic eating pattern can cause our bodies to favor the fat-storing hormones to prepare for lack of food.

By addressing underlying issues that are causing or driving the imbalance and favoring production of fat-storing hormones, not only are you fixing the real cause of the symptom, but weight loss is usually a nice side effect of just becoming healthier overall.

Other Tips for Hormone Balance

1. Get adequate sleep to repair and recover. Sleep is also important in hormone regulation, specifically cortisol.

2. Exercise to help achieve ideal estrogen ratios to minimize or prevent issues arising from estrogen dominance.

3. Increase insulin sensitivity through diet and nutrient support to lessen the negative effects of too much insulin.

4. Get properly tested for Hashimoto's by asking your doctor to check both TPO antibodies and thyroglobulin antibodies.

5. Always look upstream for why the imbalance began in the first place. What diet and lifestyle habits may have contributed to this issue, and how can you prevent that in the future?

Nutrient Therapy for Hormone Balance

Hypothyroidism and Hashimoto's

Hypothyroidism and Hashimoto's are common companions with lupus. Having suboptimal thyroid hormone levels doesn't just affect the thyroid or endocrine system. Low levels of the active thyroid hormone, T3, or inefficiencies in getting that hormone into the cells to use it affects every cell in the body. A lack of thyroid hormone leads to the foundational issue of your cells not having what they need to function, and if your cells don't work, how can anything else work? But remember, it's not enough to simply replace the missing hormones because that doesn't address the reason why they were suboptimal to begin with, hence your treatment may only be a temporary Band-Aid. In order to effectively reverse this issue to avoid the complications and symptoms of having low thyroid, you need to address the why. Your thyroid levels could be suboptimal for a number of reasons:

1. You could have an issue making thyroid hormone. Hashimoto's, the autoimmune process that causes destruction of your thyroid gland, makes it harder for your gland to produce the necessary hormones.

2. You could have an issue blocking conversion of hormone into the active form of T3 from the inactive form of T4. This can occur in places such as the liver or gut where a lot of this conversion happens. Gut issues, liver issues, or nutrient deficiencies can inhibit this process and need to be addressed to fix it.

3. You could be stressed. We know that the stress hormone cortisol can block thyroid hormone production, conversion, and uptake.

Following are some general nutrients that sometimes may need to be supplemented to support proper production, conversion, and usage of thyroid hormone.

Nutrient Support for Thyroid
Support for Hypothyroid
Selenium
Zinc
Iron
Vitamin D
Vitamin A
Nigella sativa (black cumin)

Supporting Sex Hormones

Creating or supporting balance of sex hormones really happens upstream, meaning for the most part, the how and why hormones are made, used, and balanced is a direct result of everything else going on in the body. For instance, if you have insulin resistance and are secreting high amounts of inflammatory insulin, that can impact how the sex hormones are made. The process of aromatization refers to the conversion of testosterone into estrogen. Men with insulin resistance can undergo excess aromatization and therefore become estrogen dominant due to the effects of having insulin resistance.

We even talked earlier about how issues with detoxification systems can impact the ability to effectively clear out excess hormone-creating issues such as estrogen dominance. The point is, when evaluating hormones, it's not enough to simply treat the symptoms or lab values; you must first determine if other areas of dysfunction are contributing to the imbalance and address those first. When we address other underlying factors in someone's health, their hormone symptoms or imbalances seem to fix themselves. But when the problem doesn't resolve or additional help is needed to support the body's hormone balance, a number of nutrients can assist in regaining hormonal balance. Here are a few common nutrients that are effective in assisting hormone balance.

Nutrient Support for Sex Hormones
Support for Sex Hormone Balance
Flax seed
Isoflavones
Indole-3-carbinol (I3C)
Diindolylmethane (DIM)
Fiber and other support for detox pathways

Supporting Hormones Through Menopause

When a woman goes through menopause, there is a transition of hormone production away from the ovaries and to the adrenals. This transition is a delicate balance that needs to happen smoothly or else the woman experiences the dreaded "menopause symptoms." Unfortunately, so many women just accept menopause symptoms as normal and expect it to happen to them. But it doesn't have to be that way. Remember, symptoms are telling you something is not working right. Menopause symptoms are no different. So, before you rush out and get put on hormone replacement therapy for the hot flashes and mood swings, let's talk about why this happens and what you can do about it.

Menopause is a time when a woman's ovaries stop producing hormones, her estrogen levels drop, and she stops having her monthly menses. But this doesn't mean you don't make any estrogen anymore or that your body is flawed in any way. When your ovaries stop functioning after childbearing age, the role of hormone production is turned over to another gland responsible for producing hormones, the adrenals. As you may remember from earlier chapters, the adrenal glands produce hormones, such as cortisol and adrenaline, to regulate such functions as the sleep/wake cycle and stress response. But the adrenals also make a hormone called DHEA, the precursor hormone for the main sex hormones, namely testosterone and estrogen. When you go through menopause, that hormone production relies on the adrenals to be working efficiently to supply all the cortisol the body needs and the sex hormones. If your body is under stress and your adrenals are not up to par, this creates symptoms specifically related to imbalanced hormone levels: hot flashes, night sweats, mood swings, dryness, and low libido. The standard approach to treating menopause is hormone replacement. But as we have mentioned before, just giving the body more hormones without asking or fixing why they were low to begin with is just a Band-Aid approach and one that can leave the problem under the surface to fester and cause more issues.

Due to the close nature of adrenal issues and menopause symptoms, it is common to see menopause issues lessen or resolve by addressing stress and supporting the adrenals. Make sure to get adequate sleep, practice relaxation and stress-relieving exercises daily, exercise, and use adaptogenic herbs for support.

CHAPTER ELEVEN

The Gut

Food and Nutrition for a Healthy Gut

Restricting the diet long term has a couple of major consequences: it restricts the microbiome diversity and creates more potential for immune reactions. By restricting variety in the diet, you restrict the number and types of nutrients you get and literally restrict the food sources for your microbiome, which we know is critical for a healthy immune system and overall health. Restricting the diet also increases the chances of forming new reactions to the foods you eat most often. The more exposure your immune system has to something, the more chances it has to react to it.

Immune tolerance is the immune system's ability to recognize a substance as something that is supposed to be there and not something that is foreign or harmful. Immune tolerance is something that can easily be lost but can also be regained. For example, many times people begin to lose immune tolerance to foods they eat on a regular basis, and after avoiding that food through a dietary intervention such as the elimination diet, and healing the gut, many times that food can be reintroduced back into the diet and tolerated again.

So how do you avoid losing tolerance to something in the first place? By simply not eating the same things too often. This can be achieved through something called the rotation diet. The rotation diet can simply be followed by eating only certain foods in a twenty-four-hour period and then not eating them again for four days. By rotating your favorite foods in your diet and abstaining from eating them daily, you can minimize the risk of developing a reaction from loss of tolerance.

Dietary Interventions

A number of different dietary interventions can help and address gut-specific issues. The most common recommended plans are listed below. Depending on other issues you may be experiencing, you may want to modify your dietary approach to follow one of the following food plans.

Elimination Diet

The elimination diet is a great starting place for anyone dealing with a chronic health issue. It is perfect for anyone who knows or suspects that they react to or do not tolerate a food or foods well and helps assess whether a food reaction—an allergy, an intolerance, or a sensitivity—is significantly impacting their health.

Autoimmune Paleo Diet

The AIP diet, or Autoimmune Paleo die*t*, dives deeper than the elimination diet to more specifically remove potential immune triggers from the diet and help decrease inflammation. People with a known or suspected autoimmune disease benefit from this dietary approach. While we do not specifically prescribe the AIP diet in practice but rather personalize the dietary recommendations for each individual, the general principles of the AIP diet are at the core, and following this approach is a great starting place to help get your autoimmune disease into remission.

Anti-Candida Food Plan

The anti-candida food plan is used to treat yeast or candida overgrowth and may also be helpful for dysbiosis (an overgrowth of bad bacteria) or following an elimination diet. You should consider following the anti-candida food plan if you suspect or know you have a yeast overgrowth or are experiencing gastrointestinal issues such as gas, bloating, or IBS (irritable bowel syndrome) symptoms such as changes in bowels, diarrhea, or constipation.

Low-FODMAP Food Plan

The Low-FODMAP Food Plan is more specific for people dealing with gastrointestinal symptoms, IBS, diarrhea, and constipation. It limits foods high in FODMAPS, a family of poorly absorbed, short-chain carbohydrates, which are highly fermentable in the presence of gut bacteria.

If high-FODMAP foods, such as broccoli, asparagus, onions, and garlic, cause you to bloat or cause gastrointestinal symptoms, then you should be tested for *small intestinal bacterial overgrowth* and follow the FODMAP diet to relieve symptoms and help starve the overgrowth.

Specific Carbohydrate Diet

The Specific Carbohydrate Diet eliminates complex carbohydrates, lactose, sucrose, and other inflammatory or hard-to-digest ingredients from the digestive tract to decrease inflammation and allow healing. People who have an inflammatory bowel disease, such as Crohn's or ulcerative colitis, typically do better following this dietary approach. Also, people with intolerances who lack adequate enzymes to digest well do well with this approach as a way to "give the gut a break," in a sense, from having to overwork.

While we encourage everyone with an autoimmune disease to seek out and work with an appropriate functional medicine practitioner, you can use many online resources to start with and implement these dietary interventions. It is never too soon to start implementing healthier dietary changes, even before a diagnosis.

Lifestyle for a Healthy Gut

Lifestyle, or what you do and how you do it on a regular basis, plays a significant role in gut health. Think about how much work your gut has to do on a regular basis. Every time you eat, it has to secrete the necessary enzymes, break everything down into the smallest possible components, absorb the nutrients, and process and eliminate waste all while also trying to protect you from foreign invaders, signal to you what you should and should not be eating, and repair the damage that naturally occurs through this process. So, while what you eat is very important, how and when and why you eat is just as important. Here are a few simple tips to make sure you are supporting your gut so it can support you.

Tips:

- Thoroughly chew your food. While this may sound like a no-brainer, pay attention to how many times you chew before swallowing at your next meal. You will probably be surprised to find you don't chew close to the recommended thirty times before swallowing! The simple act of better chewing your food helps you digest better, leading to less chance of food reactions as well as better ability to absorb nutrients.

- Eat with intention. Be mindful. Being in a more relaxed state when eating is helpful as your nervous system is primed for better digestion being in a parasympathetic (rest-and-digest) state. Some people may want or need to meditate or do some deep breathing before they eat to better prime their body for better digestion and absorption. Try to avoid eating when you are really stressed, or take a few minutes to relax before eating to avoid any gastrointestinal issues that may occur due to poor digestion.

- Listen to your body in terms of how it reacts to food. Do you get bloated, gassy, or uncomfortable when you eat? Do you get acid reflux or abdominal pain? Do your other symptoms such as fatigue, joint pain, brain fog, and/or skin issues get worse with eating certain foods? Get used to paying attention to your body so you get better at being able to identify what causes problems so you can avoid them.

Good Bowel Habits

How Often

How often do you have a bowel movement? While this question may seem silly or invasive, it is actually a super-important look into your gut health. How often you go number two and how it comes out can tell you a lot about what's going on inside.

First, bowel movements should be *daily, not weekly.* Many times, we get so used to our issues that they become our "normal." We have seen so many patients who think a bowel movement every three days or as little as once a week is normal because that's what they are used to!

Second, how does it come out? Is its hard bits and pieces? Smooth and easy? Or soft and loose? Do you have to run to the bathroom soon after eating? Being open with your practitioner about these sometimes-embarrassing questions can help them figure out what is going on and how to better your gut health.

Now if bowel movements aren't something you typically pay attention to, simply start by paying attention to how often you go in a typical day and keep a journal to note any changes or issues you may be having.

*Note: See the **Bristol Stool Chart** *in the tools and resources section at end of this book for more information on what to look for when evaluating bowel movements.*

Squatting Versus Sitting

Believe it or not, the human body was not designed to be in a sitting position when evacuating our bowels. The puborectalis muscle loops around the end of our bowels and the rectum, and essentially "kinks" the colon upon assuming a sitting position, just like putting a kink in the garden hose. This makes it harder for our bowels to fully evacuate and can contribute to straining.

The natural body position that favors relaxing the puborectalis muscle is squatting. By squatting, you relax this muscle and allow gravity to help empty the bowels. If you are not comfortable squatting to go number two, simply get a stool (such as the Squatty Potty) or something to put your feet on that raises the level of your knees to mimic squatting.

A Word on Fasting for Gut Health

Research has shown fasting benefits gut health and repairs the immune system. In fact, fasting for just three days acts as a "reset" for the gut and immune system. This works by essentially giving the gut a break from the constant wear and tear it experiences from constant exposure to food and other substances that are normally broken down and processed in the gut. The cells that make up the gut lining in the small intestine, where most of the breakdown and processing occurs, replace themselves every two to five days, making fasting a great way to help facilitate this natural healing process.

While you can fast in a number of ways, individual tolerance to fasting can vary widely person to person. While some people can tolerate strict water fasting, many people dealing with other chronic health issues may tolerate less extreme forms of fasting such as intermittent fasting, a modified lemonade cleanse, fasting mimicking diet, elemental diet, or simply temporarily limiting amount and variety in the diet to give the gut a break. Fasting should be done and supervised under the care of an appropriate healthcare provider.

Nutrient Therapy for a Healthy Gut

Following the 5R approach to healing the gut is a great way to make sure the underlying issues are being addressed. Following are some general nutrient recommendations for each of the sections of the 5R approach.

Nutrient Support for Gut Health	
Remove	Avoid or minimize anti-nutrient foods such as those with high lectin content, additives, preservatives, and/or heavy metals Use **activated charcoal** for binding toxins for removal Make sure you're having daily bowel movements. If needed, use **aloe vera or magnesium** as natural laxative. Coffee enemas and **ginger** can also help stimulate proper bowel movement.

Replace	*May need to replace based on symptoms and/or stool testing:* **Bile acids** **Hydrochloric acid** **Digestive enzymes**
Reinoculate	*Support a healthy microbiome by reinoculating with:* **Prebiotics** such as asparagus, banana, dandelion greens, garlic, onion, jicama, legumes **Probiotics** and probiotic foods such as fermented vegetables, kimchi, kombucha, miso, sauerkraut **Soluble fiber** such as apples, citrus fruits, strawberries, beans, peas, lentils
Repair	*Nutrients that can aid in repairing the gut lining include:* **L-glutamine** **Zinc L-carnosine** **Vitamin A** **Aloe vera** **Deglycyrrhizinated licorice** **Colostrum** **Short-chain fatty acids** as found in ghee
Rebalance	Eat a well-balanced, anti-inflammatory diet Intermittently fast for gut reset

CHAPTER TWELVE

Nutrient Deficiencies

Phytonutrients

Plant foods offer some of the best "medicine" on earth: phytonutrients. Besides giving us necessary macronutrients in terms of carbs, fiber, and proteins and micronutrients like vitamins and minerals, plants offer substances called phytonutrients to help us heal. Some of these powerful substances are things like sulforaphane from cruciferous veggies like broccoli, which is known for its anti-inflammatory and antioxidant effects.

To get the most health benefit from your food, you want to consider the importance of getting enough variety of macronutrients, micronutrients, and phytonutrients and use healthy cooking methods to better preserve their health benefits.

Importance of Variety in Diet

By eating a wide variety of foods in your diet, you not only benefit from getting a more diverse supply of nutrients, but you also minimize the negative effects of eating the same things frequently. Eating the same foods day after day can actually lead to problems with developing reactions to those foods. Many people have an issue with gluten-containing grains such as wheat because they get too much exposure to it too frequently since it is found in so many common foods people consume for breakfast, lunch, dinner, and snacks!

Rotate your favorite foods so you are not eating them every day. Choose new foods you haven't tried and try them in different ways (raw, cooked, mixed with other ingredients, etc.). Also, don't be afraid to mix and match ingredients in your favorite recipes for a new take on an old favorite.

Nutrient Therapy for General Support

Multivitamin/Multimineral

In an ideal world, a multivitamin would not be necessary. Unfortunately, in today's modern society an overwhelming majority of us are lacking sufficient intake of various nutrients. Having a good-quality multivitamin ensures that you are satisfying your vitamin and mineral requirements. It is especially important when you have lupus or any disease process that your body has everything it needs to function optimally.

Vitamin D

It is recommended that patients with lupus avoid sunlight as many tend to have photosensitivity, and sunlight can flare symptoms. This is problematic though because our greatest source of vitamin D3 is from the sun! And vitamin D3 is potentially one of the most important nutrients for regulating your immune system. Most people with chronic conditions and inflammation, especially autoimmune patients, are low in vitamin D, and this may be because the body demands more during times of inflammation and immune upregulation. Supplementation with vitamin D tends to be necessary in autoimmune patients and specifically in lupus as many people are forced to avoid the sun.

Fish Oil

Fish oil contains essential fatty acids including eicosapentaenoic acid (EPA) and docosahexaenoic acid (DHA). These omega-3 fatty acids are fundamental to help reduce inflammation in our body and have also been shown to dampen autoimmune disease. It is estimated up to 80 percent of the United States population is deficient in omega-3 fatty acids. A vegan source of omega-3 fatty acids includes algal oil.

CHAPTER THIRTEEN

Immune Balance

Balancing the Immune System

As we have discussed, a number of contributing factors can trigger and perpetuate an autoimmune tendency with the immune system. But what is actually happening in the immune system itself to cause destruction of self-tissue? Well, just like all other systems in the body, it comes down to balance and the ability to self-regulate, which is what those underlying causes interfere with.

Acute infections and tissue destruction cause your immune system to activate and stimulate production of the immune cells necessary to react and clean up the inflammation that occurs. When this is a temporary issue, the immune system temporarily upregulates production of immune cells to address this inflammatory response and then calms down and regains balance. But when the stimulus doesn't go away or the immune system can't keep up with its job of clearing out the infection or tissue damage, this inflammatory response doesn't turn off, causing chronic inflammation.

What Is Inflammation?

It's important to have a basic understanding of what inflammation is and how your immune system functions when talking about how to regain control of an imbalanced immune system as it relates to autoimmunity. Don't worry if you don't fully understand this, and feel free to skip this part or come back later.

Inflammation is basically the body's mechanism for "cleaning house." On a cellular level, white blood cells increase in the area of the body that is having tissue destruction or an infection. These white blood cells essentially "eat up" the foreign invaders or the damaged tissues and clear them out into the lymphatics. If the immune system is effective at cleaning up all the damaged tissues or pathogens, the inflammation stops and the immune system falls back into balance.

The damaged cells and/or pathogens that don't get cleared from the tissue by the immune system continue to release inflammatory chemicals to provoke inflammation to drive more and more white blood cells into that area (like calling in more troops for battle). If your body has too much going on for the immune system to effectively handle, then the inflammation continues and leads to more stress on the immune system as it tries to get rid of the bad things to restore normal function in that area. Again, inflammation itself is not the bad guy. It is a healing mechanism in the body and essential for normal healing and repair, but too much of a good thing is never a good thing, and when inflammation is left unchecked and becomes chronic, it causes damage.

When tissues are damaged or there is a foreign invader, such as a bacteria or virus, inflammatory chemicals are released in the tissue to signal the immune system to clean up the damage or toxins. The inflammatory chemicals that are released from damaged tissue or in response to pathogens stimulate the immune system and act as a signal to call in the troops for battle. This is a normal and essential role of the immune system to protect us. But when inflammation doesn't get turned off and the immune system is under constant demand, the troops start to dwindle and the body has a harder and harder time solving this issue, allowing for the problem to not only continue but sometimes exacerbate, leading to an imbalance in the functioning of the immune system.

The Delicate Balancing Act

For simplicity's sake, let's picture the immune system like a balancing scale where both sides are supposed to balance out equally. The two sides of the scale represent the different types of immune cells being produced. Although many, many more cells are actually involved, for the sake of this book, we are going to keep it simple by using Th1 (T helper 1) and Th2 (T helper 2) and Treg (T regulatory cell) to represent the cells of the immune system.

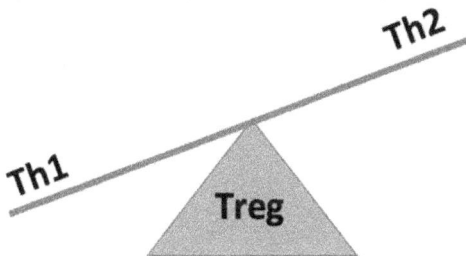

When something inflammatory happens in the body, the immune system is called into action and will temporarily shift focus toward one side of the scale. Your immune system has two parts that each work in different ways: your innate immune system and your acquired immune system. Your innate immune system is built to quickly handle and fight off any potentially harmful foreign invaders or substances, whereas your acquired immune system creates "memory cells" to aid in remembering those harmful substances it comes across to better fight them off next time. For example, if you get chicken pox, your innate immune system will recognize that virus as something that is not supposed to be there and cause an attack against it. At the same time, your acquired immune system starts to create antibodies to remember this virus so if it ever encounters it again, if you get exposed to it in the future, your immune system will remember how to fight it off so you don't end up with chicken pox or shingles. Vaccines work to simulate or stimulate an acquired immunity for the same reason.

Chronic inflammation and stress on the body create a situation where the Th1 side of the immune system is suppressed, allowing for the Th2 side to be more overactive (as pictured in the graphic). One of the important jobs of Th1 is to suppress Th17 cells, which play a major role in the tissue destruction aspect of autoimmunity. This imbalance with the immune system is not only the perfect opportunity for autoimmunity to be triggered, but also the more tissue destruction and inflammation that comes as a result of the autoimmune process, the further autoimmunity itself perpetuates. Therefore, by controlling and dampening inflammation and stress, we can better modulate and support proper balance of the immune system. This is why properly identifying and addressing sources of inflammation and stress in the body is so important in halting autoimmunity and achieving remission.

Food and Nutrition for Immune Balance

A good place to start when it comes to food and immune system balance is simply removing inflammatory and potentially immune-stimulatory foods from the diet. Following an elimination diet or autoimmune paleo protocol can assist in this process. These simple dietary changes can make a positive impact on your immune system's ability to function well and can help support balance:

Nutrition for Immune Support	
Eat	**Avoid**
Anti-inflammatory diet: AIP or elimination	Antigenic foods: foods that are reactive or cause symptoms
Low-glycemic fruits and vegetables	High-glycemic foods: higher-glycemic diets are associated with higher levels of inflammation
Foods with high-phytonutrient content: eat a rainbow of colors everyday	High-lectin content: consider low-lectin if sensitive
Adequate omega-3 fatty acids: omega-3s are anti-inflammatory and can support immune balance	Trans-fats, pro-inflammatory omega-6s and inflammatory or highly processed oils
Gluten-free and dairy-free	Excessive salt intake: associated with upregulation of the tissue-destructive Th17 cells Coffee/caffeine shown to shift toward Th2 dominance

Lifestyle for Maintaining Immune Balance

"We are what we repeatedly do.
Excellence, then, is not an act, but a habit."

—*Will Durant*

As we've discussed in the previous sections, creating a healthy lifestyle revolves around identifying and modifying the things we do on a daily basis that are sabotaging our health and further perpetuating chronic disease.

Lifestyle Tips

1. Get adequate sleep. Sleep deprivation, even mild, can elevate inflammatory markers.

2. Stop smoking. Smoking or vaping nicotine is toxic, leads to increased inflammation and oxidative stress, and is an immune system irritant. Nicotine increases cortisol levels and blood pressure and can increase risk of heart attack. Don't sabotage your health.

3. Exercise. Make sure not to overdo it as strenuous exercise can perpetuate leaky gut and contribute to stress in the body.

4. Incorporate daily stress management techniques. When it comes to supporting the immune system, we cannot stress enough the importance of stress management in not only healing but also maintaining remission. Remember, chronic stress is pro-inflammatory, meaning it contributes immune system overactivation and leads to flares of the disease. Thus, you should make it a priority to learn ways to cope with stress and avoid as many external stressors as possible.

Photosensitivity

Sensitivity to the sun can be devastating as you have to plan your day around avoiding the sun or suffer the consequences. The sun's UV rays can cause skin damage and trigger an immune flare-up and symptoms. In sun-sensitive individuals, sun exposure can mean painful sunburns, rashes, aches and pains, and fatigue even after short stints in the sun.

So how can you avoid/minimize UV exposure?

1. Cover up! Wear a hat, long sleeves, an umbrella, and gloves.

2. Avoid the sun between 11 a.m. and 3 p.m. as this is when the sun's rays are strongest.

3. Use a natural broad-spectrum sunscreen daily.

4. Be aware of the effects of indoor lighting as indoor fluorescent lights can also create problems in some sensitive people. Don't be afraid to discuss with your employer, etc.

5. Be aware of things that may increase your sensitivity to the sun:

   - Certain drugs can contribute to or increase photosensitivity, such as certain antifungal drugs, antihistamines, oral contraceptives, non-steroidal anti-inflammatory drugs (NSAIDs like ibuprofen and naproxen), antibiotics, oral diabetes drugs, diuretics, and tricyclic antidepressants. The same is true of the herbal remedy St. John's wort, which is taken for depression, anxiety, and PMS.

   - Consuming foods such as celery, dill, fennel, figs, lime, parsley, and wild carrots can increase sun sensitivity.

- Topical scents and essential oils like bergamot, bitter orange, lavender, lemon verbena, musk, rosemary, and sandalwood can make your skin more reactive to the sun.

- Check skin care products for ingredients such as glycolic acid, salicylic acid, and Retin-A. Each of these agents strips the outer layer of the skin, making the skin more sensitive to the sun. Plus, the chemical benzoyl peroxide, which is in many over-the-counter acne products, can cause photosensitivity.

The supplemental herb Polypodium leucotomos may help with skin protection to reduce symptoms or flares with sun exposure. This plant extract has been shown to protect against free radical damage in the skin like what can occur from UV exposure.

It is really important for sun-sensitive people to supplement with oral vitamin D to ensure adequate amounts for immune support.

Nutrient Therapy for Immune Balance

Nutrient Support for Immune Balance	
Th1 Specific Support	Zinc Berberine HCL Chinese skullcap Sulforaphane Ginger
Th2 Modulation Support	NAC (n-acetyl-l-cysteine) Astragalus Quercetin
Treg and Overall Immune Support	Vitamin D3 Vitamin A + carotenoids Zinc Omega-3 fatty acids Turmeric (Curcumin) Resveratrol Black ginger Quercetin Andrographis paniculata
Support for Flare-Up	*Increase dosage of above support and add in additional:* Glutathione Turmeric

CHAPTER FOURTEEN

Chronic Infections

Food and Nutrition for Fighting Infections

When it comes to food and nutrition for fighting infections, often what you avoid is more important than what you eat. Overall following a low-glycemic diet and avoiding sugars and foods that exacerbate symptoms can help with combating infections and keeping inflammation down.

The **anti-candida** and **Low-FODMAP** Food Plans are used to treat overgrowths and dysbiosis in the gut. These food plans specifically eliminate foods that are known to "feed" the bacteria or yeast and helps to starve them out. Many people with gastrointestinal overgrowths feel better simply following these dietary changes.

Lifestyle for Preventing Infection

While we cannot truly avoid exposure to potentially infectious organisms, we can minimize the risk of developing an infection and can support our body's natural ability to defend us and fight off the foreign invaders.

Unfortunately, we can't live in a bubble, and the cold truth is, we are constantly exposed to a multitude of potentially harmful bacteria, viruses, yeast, and parasites on a daily basis. They are in our food, water, and air, living on and in us, and we exist in a symbiotic relationship with these natural organisms. In fact, our own human cells are outnumbered by bacteria by about ten to one! So why aren't we constantly sick? Because not all microbial organisms are harmful. In fact, many are even known to be beneficial, and we rely on them for optimal health. But when things become imbalanced and we have too many "bad guys," our immune systems are not equipped to fight them off; that's when problems arise.

Protecting Our Microbiome

We discussed the gut microbiome in depth earlier, but did you know that each area of the body has a different microbiome? The skin, mouth, nose, colon, and vagina all have unique microbiomes, and disruption of this delicate balance can cause system-wide issues. Our exposure to the world is what helps us build our microbiomes, and in today's day and age of over sanitization efforts, we are disrupting our natural microbial ecosystem. So here are some tips for protecting your microbiome:

1. Avoid herbicides, pesticides, overuse of hand sanitizer, bleach, and "disinfecting" agents and opt for more natural and organic products.

2. Have young kids? Let them play in the dirt, let them get dirty; it will build their immune system and help them get sick less often.

3. Ensure that you are having regular bowel movements daily. Not moving your bowels daily can lead to problems in the microbiome as waste and toxins aren't efficiently cleared out, leaving room for harboring the perfect environment for dysbiotic or potentially harmful organisms to thrive. Start by making sure you are drinking enough water every day. Consuming fiber-rich foods and practicing stress management techniques that support the parasympathetics also help keep bowels moving.

4. Avoid overuse of antibiotics. This is huge. All too often antibiotics are being readily used for every little infection, which is creating an epidemic of antibiotic-resistant super bugs. Avoid antibiotics for minor colds or infections when possible.

5. Avoid the use of too many topical/cosmetic products. Using too many chemicals on our skin leads to toxic exposure and interferes with our skin's natural ability to take care of itself.

6. Maintain good oral hygiene and have regular checkups with your dentist to check for any infections or sources of inflammation.

Gingivitis and Periodontal Disease

One of the most common places for hidden infections is the mouth. There's a lot of evidence that oral bacteria can lead to systemic infection, and poor oral hygiene has been connected to chronic inflammation and a whole host of chronic health conditions. Maintaining good oral hygiene can have an overall positive effect on your health and help you achieve remission.

Good Oral Hygiene Tips:

- Floss daily.

- Brush teeth two times a day for more than two minutes.

- Avoid sugary foods and drinks.

- Avoid toxic toothpaste and oral hygiene products.

- Use activated charcoal toothpaste. (Activated charcoal binds to toxins and chemicals and prevents them from being absorbed in the body. Besides being a great detoxifier and helping to remove toxic waste from the body, it also is a great natural whitening agent for your teeth. But even more so, charcoal can help with pH balance in the mouth and support proper balance of your oral microbiome.)

- Consider using an oral probiotic to support the mouth microbiome.

Nutrient Therapy for Infections

The term *infection* refers to an invasion of disease-causing agents and the body's reaction to those agents and the toxins they produce. The body is very intelligent when it comes to infections and protecting us from harm. But what happens when our immune system isn't able to effectively do its job? The following chart outlines important herbs and natural agents that can effectively help eradicate different types of infections. This is by no means a complete list but rather guidance for those suffering from different types of infections as to what has been effective in treating these different types of infections.

Herbal Treatments

Herbal Treatments for Infections		
Bacterial Infections	**Fungal Infections**	**Parasitic Infections**
Garlic	Oregano	Black walnut
Goldenseal	Thyme	Wormwood
Berberine	Garlic	Bitterwood
Uva ursi	Goldenseal	Garlic
Oregano	Probiotics & saccharomyces boulardii	Goldenseal
Grapefruit seed extract		Oregano
Thyme		Olive leaf
		Citrus seed extract
		Thyme
Upper Respiratory Infection	**Viral Infections**	**Urinary Tract Infections**
Vitamin D	Monolaurin	D-mannose
Vitamin C with flavonoids	L-Lysine	Cranberry
N-acetylcysteine	Cats claw	Uva ursi
Andrographis	Olive leaf	Berberine
Licorice root		Marshmallow root
Umckaloabo		Bladderwrack
Olive leaf extract		Celery seed extract
Elderberry (liquid)		
Garlic (freeze-dried)		

Chronic Sinusitis

Chronic sinus inflammation or issues such as congestion, postnasal drip, and excess mucus production can commonly be traced back to an underlying infection in the sinus cavities. To address this, use a nasal-irrigation tool and antimicrobials directly in the sinus cavities. A nasal-irrigation tool, such as a neti pot, is an easy way to help clear out the sinuses and help fight off underlying infections. Always make sure to use clean, distilled water (not tap water) and add in an antimicrobial such as colloidal silver to increase effectiveness and combat infections and inflammation.

If you are new to nasal irrigation, it may seem weird or uncomfortable at first, but as you practice, it becomes easier and can soon be your best friend for all your sinus issues!

Sinusitis

Nasal irrigation can be a great tool for helping clear and soothe the sinus cavities but can also help eradicate infectious agents that may contribute to overall inflammation and immune activation.

What you need:	Nasal cleansing (neti) pot
	~1/2 tsp. of uniodized salt
	~ 8oz. distilled water
	Additionally can add:
	1-2 caps of berberine to saline
	1-2 drops of tea tree oil to saline (may be irritating) colloidal silver to saline

Directions:	1.	Prepare saline solution and fill nasal cleansing pot
	2.	Place spout of pot up to nostril
	3.	Lean over sink and tilt your head away from pot
	4.	The water will enter higher nostril and come out the opposite nostril
	5.	Stop and blow your nose before switching to opposite side with remaining solution

Nicole's Life in Remission: Patient Plan and Resolution

Nicole followed the elimination diet to clean up her diet, remove inflammatory foods, and identify food sensitivities. We started her on some anti-inflammatory nutraceuticals such as turmeric, glutathione, and omega-3s as well as starting her on a high dose of vitamin D3.

To address her leaky gut and heal it, we killed the bad bacteria and repopulated it with good probiotics and prebiotics to rebalance the microbiome.

We supported her immune system through diet, lifestyle, nutrition, and stress management with the principles in this book. We focused on stabilizing her blood sugar to support her adrenals so she could sleep better.

Gradually, we worked on each of these areas one at a time and found what worked for her body, monitoring her labs to watch the changes and modify the plan as we went along. The first victory was getting her to sleep through the night within the first month, which was the first time she had gotten good sleep in months.

Taking small steps over time, Nicole started to feel like herself again.

By the end of six months, Nicole was off all her meds.

No more Prednisone.

No more Plaquenil.

No more antidepressants, allergy meds, or pain pills.

She was sleeping through the night. And had stable energy through the day.

She wasn't having the headaches or joint pains.

Her dry mouth and eyes were improving, and her brain fog was gone.

She was back to work full time again and back to living her normal life for the first time in years.

At our year follow-up, she was still off all her meds, and all her labs were continuing to improve while her antibodies were lowered. All her specialists were very impressed and kept telling her to "keep doing whatever you're doing." She is loving her newfound life and feels empowered to know how to control her health, so it doesn't control her.

CHAPTER FIFTEEN

Resources

Next Steps

The information in this book is designed to give you a better understanding of lupus and autoimmunity and provide information about steps you can start taking to improve your health and work toward remission. These resources can help you identify and begin to implement healthy changes so you can start taking your health into your own hands. If you found this information valuable, we would love for you to share it with someone you care about and help get the word out by leaving us a review on Amazon.

One-on-One Coaching

We offer one-on-one coaching programs for those needing or wanting more personalized support and specific recommendations. We work with individuals on identifying and addressing their unique underlying causes of autoimmunity to help them regain their health and achieve remission. This is a great opportunity to get answers specific to you and the guidance and accountability to reach your health goals. We work with people virtually around the world, so no matter where you are, you too can get the help you need. For more information about working with us one-on-one and to apply visit caplanhealthinstitute.com.

At-Home Course

For more help implementing the information in this book you can check out our online Lupus Solution Course at caplanhealthinstitute.com. With this online program, you can go at your own pace learning the tools and steps to help you better understand your health and what you need to do to finally feel better. This course consists of 8 weekly modules with lots of videos and handouts to help you learn how to take control of your life.

Connect Online

We also encourage you to join our Lupus and Autoimmunity Support Group (Caplan Health Institute) Facebook page to connect with others going through the same health journey and for a chance to find support and get some of your questions answered.

Tools and Resources

This section provides resources that will help you on your health journey. Use these worksheets to take notes and keep track of new things you learn and discover about yourself as you go through the book. These tools can help you create your own customized workbook to give you a better idea of where you need to start implementing changes to take control of your health.

For example, if your goal is to have better energy by getting better sleep, you may want to focus on underlying issues with blood sugar or adrenals, which could be causing the sleep problems and therefore interfering with your energy throughout the day.

*You can print these resources by downloading our free Lupus Solution Workbook
by visiting www.caplanhealthinstitute.com/thelupussolutionbook.

Notes

Blood Sugar/Insulin

My symptoms associated with this area

Dietary and lifestyle changes to address this

Adrenals/Cortisol

My symptoms associated with this area

Dietary and lifestyle changes to address this

Thyroid and Hormone Balance

My symptoms associated with this area

Dietary and lifestyle changes to address this

Gut Issues and Infections

My symptoms associated with this area

Dietary and lifestyle changes to address this

Toxins and Chemicals
My symptoms associated with this area
Dietary and lifestyle changes to address this

Immune Imbalances
My symptoms associated with this area
Dietary and lifestyle changes to address this

Daily Blood Sugar and Blood Pressure Log

Date	Blood Sugar Morning/Fasting	Blood Sugar Evening/ Non-Fasting	Blood Pressure	Notes

Important Lab Panels

Metabolic chemistry panel

Urinalysis

CBC with differentials and platelets

Iron and anemia markers

Hypothyroidism and Hashimoto's antibodies

Fasting insulin and hemoglobin A1c

Homocysteine and MTHFR status

Hs-CRP (high sensitivity c-reactive protein)

ESR (erythrocyte sedimentation rate)

Fibrinogen

Complement levels (C3 and C4)

HLA-DR2 and HLA-DR3

Celiac testing

Syphilis VDRL

Antiphospholipid and anticardiolipin antibodies

ANA with titer

Anti-double-stranded DNA antibody

Anti-Sm antibody

Anti-Ro/SSA and anti-La/SSB

Anti-RNP antibody

Elimination Diet

Foods to Avoid	Foods to Eat
Grains (wheat, barley, rye, spelt, emmer, farro, triticale, kamut, corn)	**All vegetables** (except nightshades)
Gluten-free grains (oats, rice, millet, quinoa, teff, buckwheat, amaranth, arrowroot, sorghum, tapioca)	**Starchy vegetables** (squash, plantain, sweet potato, yam, root vegetables [parsnip, rutabaga])
Dairy (butter, cheese, cottage cheese, cream, yogurt, ice cream, milk, whey)	**Fruits** (all fruits in moderation)
Soy and soybean products (edamame, miso, soy sauce, tamari, tempeh, tofu, soy milk, textured vegetable protein)	**Plant proteins and legumes** (beans, peas, lentils, chickpeas and hummus, protein powder [pea, hemp])
Animal proteins (beef, eggs, pork, shellfish, processed meats)	**Animal proteins** (wild-caught fish, wild game [buffalo, lamb, etc.], protein powder [collagen])
Peanuts and peanut butter	**Nuts and seeds** (except peanuts)
Fats and oils (butter, corn oil, cottonseed oil, margarine, mayonnaise, peanut oil, shortening, soybean oil)	**Fats and oils** (coconut oil, avocado oil, olive oil, ghee, olives, avocado, coconut cream, grapeseed oil, safflower oil, sunflower oil, walnut oil)
Nightshades (tomato and tomato products [salsa, tomato sauce], all peppers, eggplant, potato)	**Herbs and seasonings** (just look for added ingredients such as: sugars, food coloring, preservatives, etc.)
Beverages (coffee and caffeine products, alcohol, fruit juices)	**Beverages** (water, non-dairy milk alternatives, herbal tea)

Sleep Hygiene Checklist

Use this list to see if there are any areas of your sleep hygiene that need to be improved/modified to achieve better sleep.

___ Keep a sleep diary (track quality, quantity, and any issues)

___ Maintain a regular sleep schedule daily

___ Go to bed around the same time nightly

___ Wake up around the same time every morning

___ Sleep on a comfortable mattress

___ Pick a supportive pillow for your sleeping style

___ Control light exposure (from clocks, windows, etc.) or use sleep mask

___ Have good air circulation, use fan if needed

___ Use an air purifier to minimize allergens

___ Use apps on electronic devices to remove blue light at least a few hours before bed

___ Remove electronic devices from bedroom

___ Turn phone on airplane mode if near bed or using as alarm

___ Finish eating 2-3 hours before bedtime (unless a snack is needed for blood sugar reasons)

___ Exercise regularly (at least 3 hours before bedtime or best if in the morning)

___ Avoid caffeine, nicotine, and alcohol

___ Practice belly breathing and visualization or meditation to fall asleep if needed

___ Take an Epsom salt bath before bed for sleep

___ Use an essential oil diffuser with lavender

The Bristol Stool Chart is a great way to quickly see what your bowel movements may be telling you.

The Bristol Stool Chart

	Looks like	Consistency	Indicates
Type 1		Separate hard lumps	Very constipated
Type 2		Lumpy and sausage like	Slightly constipated
Type 3		Sausage shaped with cracks in the surface	Normal
Type 4		A smooth, soft sausage or snake	Normal
Type 5		Soft blobs with clear-cut edges	Lacking fibre
Type 6		Mushy consistency with ragged edges	Inflammation
Type 7		Liquid consistency with no solid pieces	Inflammation

Image Source: The Conversation